14th Edition
Internal Medicine Review Core Curriculum

Book 5 of 5

Topics in this volume:

General Internal Medicine

Neurology

Dermatology

Authored by Robert A. Hannaman, MD
with Candace Mitchell, MD and J. Thomas Cross, Jr., MD, MPH, FACP

Disclaimers

CONTENT: The primary purpose of this activity is educational. Medicine and accepted standards of care are constantly changing. We at MedStudy do our best to review and include in this activity accurate discussions of the standards of care, methods of diagnosis, and selection of treatments. However, the authors/presenters, editors, advisors, and publisher—and all other parties involved with the preparation of this work—disclaim any guarantee that the information contained in this activity and its associated materials is in every respect accurate or complete. MedStudy further disclaims any and all liability for damages and claims that may result from the use of information or viewpoints presented. We recommend you confirm the information contained in this activity and in any other educational material with current sources of medical knowledge whenever considering actual clinical presentations or treating patients.

ABIM. For over 20 years, MedStudy has excelled in determining and teaching what a clinically competent Internal Medicine physician should know. The American Board of Internal Medicine (ABIM) tests this exact same pool of knowledge. MedStudy's expertise, demonstrated by the superb pass rate of those who use it in their studies, is in the actual "teaching" of this knowledge in a clear, learner-friendly manner that results in a stronger knowledge base, improved clinical skills, and better Board results. Although what we teach is in sync with what the Boards test, MedStudy has no affiliation with the ABIM, and our authors, editors and reviewers have no access to ABIM exam content. Our material is developed as original work by MedStudy physician authors, with additional input from expert contributors, based on their extensive backgrounds in professional medical education. This content is designed to include subject matter typically tested in certification and recertification exams as outlined in the ABIM's publicly available exam blueprints but makes no use of, and divulges no details of, ABIM's proprietary exam content.

A note on editorial style: MedStudy follows a standardized approach to the naming of diseases, using the non-possessive form when the proper name of a disease is followed by a common noun. So you will see phrasing such as "This patient would warrant workup for Crohn disease" (as opposed to "Crohn's disease"). Possessive form will be used, however, when an entity is referred to solely by its proper name without a following common noun. An example of this would be "The symptoms are classic for Crohn's." Styles used in today's literature can be highly arbitrary, some using possessive and some not, but we believe consistency is important. It has become nearly obsolete to use the possessive form in terminology such as Lou Gehrig's disease, Klinefelter's syndrome, and others. *The AMA Manual of Style*, *JAMA*, and *Scientific Style and Format* are among the publications that are now promoting and using the non-possessive form. We concur with this preference.

MEDSTUDY®
P.O. Box 38148
Colorado Springs, Colorado 80937
(800) 841-0547

MedStudy®

IM INTERNAL MEDICINE REVIEW
CORE CURRICULUM

14th EDITION

Authored by Robert A. Hannaman, MD
with Candace Mitchell, MD

GENERAL INTERNAL MEDICINE

Many thanks to General Internal Medicine Advisors:

Douglas S. Paauw, MD, MACP
Professor of Medicine
Rathmann Family Foundation Endowed Chair
for Patient-Centered Clinical Education
Head, General Internal Medicine
Division of Internal Medicine
University of Washington School of Medicine
Seattle, WA

Allen R. Friedland, MD, FACP, FAAP
Medicine-Pediatrics Residency Program Director
Christiana Care Health System
Newark, DE

Kristin L. Kaelber, MD, PhD
Instructor of Medicine and Pediatrics
Case Western Reserve University
Cleveland, OH

Table of Contents
General Internal Medicine

PHARMACOLOGY

PHARMACOKINETICS

Absorption

First-pass effect: Oral drugs are absorbed via the GI tract and pass into the portal vein, which goes to the liver. Drugs metabolized by the liver will then undergo "first-pass" metabolism. These drugs require a much higher oral dose to be as effective as a parenteral dose of the same medicine. Common drugs that undergo first-pass effect:

1) Opiate-related: Meperidine, morphine, and naloxone
2) Calcium antagonists: Nifedipine, verapamil, and diltiazem
3) Some beta-blockers: Labetalol, metoprolol, and propranolol
4) Tricyclic antidepressants
5) Benzodiazepines (BDZs)
6) Anticonvulsants: Valproic acid and phenytoin
7) NSAIDs: Ibuprofen, ketoprofen, naproxen, and indomethacin
8) Other: Cyclophosphamide, theophylline, warfarin, and metronidazole

Some drugs require an acidic environment for absorption—especially the azole antifungals (except fluconazole and voriconazole) and thyroid hormone. These drugs should not be used with H_2 blockers or proton pump inhibitors (PPIs). PPIs can also block calcium absorption.

A very important interaction that interferes with absorption occurs when cations (calcium and iron supplements or antacids containing magnesium and aluminum) combine with thyroid hormone or quinolones.

Distribution

Volume of distribution (V) [Know]: This is the effective volume for determining the total amount of drug in the body and for determining the loading dose. The total amount of drug in the body (D_T) is equal to the volume x concentration:

$$D_T = V (C_p)$$

So the volume of distribution is:

$$V = D_T/C_p$$

V = the volume of distribution. This is the apparent volume into which the drug is dispersed. C_p is the concentration of the drug in the plasma. If the tissues hold more drug than the plasma at equilibrium, "V" will be large. Rule of thumb: If the drug is dosed at each half-life, the total amount of drug (D_T) is double the maintenance dose.

Note that the loading dose does not depend on excretion capability! The loading dose in a patient with renal failure is the same as that in a healthy patient; but if the drug is cleared by the kidney, the subsequent maintenance dose will be very different.

Excretion

Drugs excreted mainly by the liver include all of those mentioned above under first-pass effect.

In a person with cirrhosis, the decreased first-pass effect increases the effective bioavailability of the above drugs. Clearance is also decreased, so the effective dose of a drug may be very small.

Meperidine is metabolized by the liver to normeperidine, which is an active metabolite causing CNS stimulation (including seizures). Normeperidine is cleared by the kidney. So carefully watch a patient with hepatic or renal dysfunction when on meperidine!

First-Order Kinetics

First-order kinetics: The rate at which a drug is cleared is independent of the drug concentration. After one half-life, the drug level in the body will be only half of the initial level. It is possible to determine the half-life by checking 2 blood levels at a certain interval (between doses).

As seen in Table 10-1, 5 half-lives after a patient is started on a first-order drug without a loading dose, the drug level will be 97% of steady state. Also, if a first-order drug is stopped, the drug will be 97% gone after 5 half-lives. So, when starting patients on a medication with no loading dose, usually wait 3 to 5 half-lives before rechecking the blood level to see if you need to adjust the dosage.

Drug Interactions

Note

There are thousands of drug interactions, but several are very serious—and thus frequently on the Boards. We will cover some of the most serious ones here.

Table 10-1: Half-Lives	
# of Half-lives	**Percent of Steady State**
1	50
2	75
3	87.5
4	93.75
5	96.875

Table 10-2: Warfarin Interactions	
Most Severe	**Possible**
TMP/SMX	Quinolones
Erythromycin	Omeprazole
Amiodarone	Clarithromycin
Propafenone	Azithromycin
Azole antifungals	Prednisone
Metronidazole	Acetaminophen (> 1.5 g/d)

Warfarin Interactions

Table 10-2 outlines the most important warfarin interactions that result in increased INR (international normalized ratio). Especially know that trimethoprim/sulfamethoxazole (TMP/SMX) can markedly raise the INR within the first few days of therapy. TMP/SMX both displaces warfarin from protein-binding sites and decreases warfarin metabolism. However, any antibiotic can affect the INR without affecting warfarin metabolism by decreasing vitamin-producing bacteria in the intestine.

Natural products with the potential to enhance the anticoagulant effect of warfarin include glucosamine, ginkgo, garlic, feverfew, and dong quai.

Drugs that Cause Hyperkalemia

ACE inhibitors, ARBs, spironolactone and other potassium-sparing diuretics, and heparin can cause severe hyperkalemia. The risk is far greater when several of these drugs are combined (as seen in the treatment of heart failure). Trimethoprim can cause hyperkalemia by blocking amiloride-sensitive channels in the renal tubule. The risk is greatest in the elderly and with use of high-dose TMP/SMX.

Statin Interactions

The most life-threatening reaction to a statin is rhabdomyolysis. The risk is much greater when statins are combined with drugs that slow their metabolism. The drugs that affect statin hepatic metabolism are fibrates, erythromycin, cyclosporine, azole antifungals, protease inhibitors, verapamil, diltiazem, and amiodarone. Grapefruit juice will also markedly raise the blood levels of some statins by inhibiting initial hepatic metabolism. Lovastatin and simvastatin are most affected; and pravastatin is least affected (because it is metabolized by the kidneys). The most common side effect of statins is myalgias.

Other Interactions / Side Effects to Know

Know:

• Rosiglitazone and pioglitazone cause edema, worsening congestive heart failure (CHF), and weight gain.

• Dihydropyridines (nifedipine, amlodipine) cause peripheral edema and constipation.
• SSRIs cause hyponatremia, sexual dysfunction, and may cause platelet dysfunction.
• Topiramate causes non-anion gap acidosis and kidney stones.
• Hydrochlorothiazide causes low K^+, high Ca^+, low Na^+, and high uric acid.
• St. John's Wort increases metabolism of statins, cyclosporin, some HIV/AIDS drugs, and oral contraceptives ($\rightarrow$ treatment failure).
• NSAIDs increase risk of symptomatic CHF in patients at risk for coronary artery disease (CAD).
• Bisphosphonates can cause muscle and joint pain.
• PPIs may inhibit antiplatelet activity of clopidogrel.

STATISTICS

SENSITIVITY AND SPECIFICITY

The Bayesian 4 Square

Note: T = true, F = false, P = positive, N = negative

Know statistics perfectly!

To make sense of the 4 square used in answering sensitivity and specificity questions, we will go over Figure 10-1. Let's assume we have a group of cattle being tested for a deadly disease. They go through the testing station on the left and are directed to either the upper corral if their test is positive or the lower corral if their test is negative. All cattle are then driven across the corral to the right; but this disease is so deadly, all the diseased cattle die before they get to the far right of the corral. So we are left with 4 sets of cattle. The 4 square is very useful in determining sensitivity, specificity, and positive and negative predictive values.

Sensitivity and specificity try to account for those with (sensitivity) disease and those without (specificity) the disease.

Sensitivity takes into account only those who have the disease. Sensitivity = true positives (# of patients with disease who test positive) divided by the total # of patients with disease (those who test positive plus the false negatives). Sensitivity = TP/(TP + FN) (Figure 10-1).

A good screening test should try to approach 100% but usually does not because there are some patients who have the disease but do not test positive (false negatives).

Specificity takes into account only those who do not have the disease. Specificity = true negatives (# of patients without disease who test negative) divided by the total # of patients without the disease (those who test negative plus the false positives): Specificity = TN/(TN + FP).

A good confirmatory test should try to approach 100% but usually does not succeed—because some without the disease will test positive (false positives).

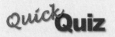

Quick Quiz

- Define first-order kinetics.
- How long should you wait before rechecking a blood level for a drug that follows first-order kinetics?
- You have invented a test that is 90% sensitive and 95% specific for screening of breast cancer. If you tested 100 women with known breast cancer, how many would the test say have breast cancer (true positives)?
- Be able to fill in a 4 square and quickly determine sensitivity, specificity, PPV, and NPV.
- Which of the following take into account disease prevalence: sensitivity, specificity, PPV, NPV.

To help remember: Note that sensitivity takes into account only those who have the disease, and specificity takes into account only those who do not have the disease. This means that sensitivity and specificity are independent of the prevalence (percentage) of the population with the disease!

The "positive predictive value" (PPV) of a diagnostic test is the probability of disease in a patient given a positive test—i.e., PPV = P(disease | positive test). To figure this, you take into account the numbers of both the true positives and the false positives. This combination does reflect prevalence. The positive predictive value is generally higher with conditions that are more prevalent (common) than those conditions that are less prevalent (rare), given the same sensitivity and specificity of a test. The formula is PPV = TP/(TP + FP). This makes sense: true positives divided by all those who test positive! If a disease is rare, even if the sensitivity and specificity are high, the false positives may greatly outnumber the true positives, making the chance of having the disease with a positive test (PPV) much less. This is one of the main factors used to determine whether a screening program is feasible.

The "negative predictive value" (NPV) of a diagnostic test is the probability of not having a disease given a negative test; i.e., NPV = P(no disease | negative test). Using the 4 square, the formula is TN/(TN + FN). NPV, like PPV, reflects the disease prevalence. The negative predictive value is generally higher with conditions that are less prevalent (rare) than those conditions that are more prevalent (common), given the same sensitivity and specificity of a test.

Tips:

- Note that in all the above (sensitivity, specificity, PPV, NPV), the "Trues" go in the numerator (on top).
- PPV deals with nothing but positives; NPV deals with nothing but negatives.

The prevalence (or prior/pretest probability) is merely the fraction of the population who has the disease. This is (Total with disease)/Total, or (TP + FN) / (TP + FN) + (FP + TN).

Not all the data may be given in a question asking you to find sensitivity, specificity, PPV, NPV; it is very

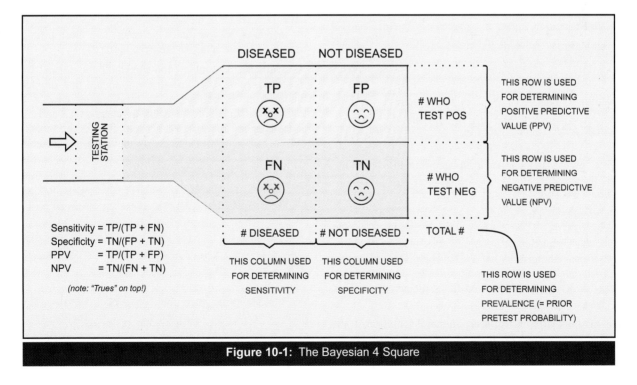

Figure 10-1: The Bayesian 4 Square

Table 10-3

	Disease	No Disease	Total
Abn tests	TP	FP	TP + FP
Nl tests	FN	TN	FN + TN
Total	TP + FN	FP + TN	

Table 10-4

I. Sketch this first:

	With	Without	Total
Abn tests			
Nl tests			
Total			

Table 10-5

II. Based on the given information:

	With	Without	Total
Abn tests	1	3	13,000
Nl tests	2	4	987,000
Total	5,000	995,000	1,000,000

Note that the 5,000 and 995,000 are the denominators in the sensitivity and specificity equations!

Table 10-6

III. Calculations

	With	Without	Total
Abn tests	4,950	8,050	13,000
Nl tests	50	986,950	987,000
Total	5,000	995,000	1,000,000

useful to use Table 10-3 in its stripped-down form (Table 10-4). You insert the given values and then calculate for the blank spaces!

The "givens" in the following example are filled in. When all the spaces are filled in, the question is easily answered. Know this stuff!

Example: Incidence of cancer is 1/200 in a population. In a test under consideration, if sensitivity = 99% and the frequency of abnormal tests in the population is 1.3%, what is the ratio of false positives to true positives—and is this a good screening test? To solve, first draw the Table 10-4 and fill in the given numbers. This gives us Table 10-5.

If the population is not given, assume 1 million. 1/200 incidence gives 5,000 total persons with cancer. 0.013 x 1 million gives 13,000 total abnormal tests.

Then just subtract to find the number without cancer (995,000) and the number of normal tests (987,000). Note that the 5,000 and 995,000 are the denominators in the sensitivity and specificity equations!

Then we find the other blanks in the order shown 1, 2, 3, and 4. Blank (1) is the only one requiring thought:

Sensitivity = TP/(TP + FN) or 0.99 = TP/5,000

So: TP = 4,950.

The others are found by subtraction (Table 10-6).

Once you have the entire matrix filled in, you can solve any problem, provided there is enough information. In this example, PPV = TP/(TP + FP) = 38%—not a good percentage for a screening test! If data given to solve the problem are insufficient, it will become apparent when you are unable to fill in all the blanks.

What happens if you change the criteria for what is called a normal test? If you increase the range for what is normal, you will get more negative tests—both true negatives and false negatives. This will decrease the sensitivity while increasing the specificity.

Why is this? Assume we did this for the previous example. Because the numbers of people with and without the disease (prevalence) remain the same, the denominators in the sensitivity and specificity equations remain the same—but the numerators change. In the sensitivity equation, the numerator decreases (decreased TP due to increased FN), so sensitivity decreases; i.e., fewer of those with the disease are found by the test. In the specificity equation, the numerator increases, so specificity increases; i.e., those testing negative are less likely to have the disease. In the specificity equation, the numerator increases, so specificity increases; i.e., those testing negative are less likely to have the disease.

As a quick tip, think of the threshold for normal on the test as being the line in the 4 square that divides the top from the bottom: As the threshold increases, the line rises, indicating decreasing numbers of TP and FP and increasing numbers of FN and TN. As the threshold decreases, the line goes lower, indicating increasing positives and decreasing negatives. Because the denominator in the sensitivity and specificity formulas stay the same, just see what happens to TP and TN. If TP increases, sensitivity increases. If TN increases, specificity increases.

You will also see that anytime the test normals are redefined, sensitivity will increase at the expense of specificity and vice-versa.

As disease prevalence and incidence decrease, the number of false positives increases while the number of false negatives decreases—so the ratio of false positives to false negatives increases. This occurs because there

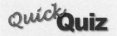

- You read that a study shows a new treatment for lung cancer improves survival by 60% and the *P* value for the study is 0.2. Based on these results, would you recommend this treatment?

- You read that a study shows a newer treatment for lung cancer improves survival by 5%, and the 95% confidence interval for the study is 1.6 to 4.9. Assuming treatments have the same side effects, would it be worthwhile to consider the new treatment?

is no change in the sensitivity or specificity of the diagnostic test.

Sensitivity, specificity, PPV, and NPV can also be interpreted from diagrams such as these:

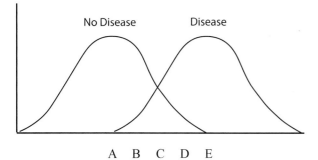

This chart shows test performance for a diagnostic test in 2 populations, 1 with the disease and 1 without.

Remember that sensitivity = [True positives/(True positives + False negatives)]. Point A would have no false negatives, since all of the group with the disease would have a value greater than A. Thus, Point A has the best sensitivity. Point A also has the best false-negative value. Point E has no false positives and would have the best specificity and the best positive predictive value.

P Value and Confidence Intervals

The *P* value is a way of expressing a study's statistical significance. Suppose a randomized trial compares 2 drugs and concludes that Drug A is better than Drug B. The smaller the *P* value, the more confident we can be that drug A really is better than drug—and that this is not simply a chance occurrence. Thus, if a study has a *P* value of 0.05, the likelihood that the results are due to chance is only 1 in 20 (= 5%; or *P* = 0.05). *P* values of less than 0.05—such as 0.01 or 0.001—imply even greater statistical significance. A *P* value ≤ 0.05 is considered statistically significant.

The above (*P* < 0.05, ha!) is probably all you need to know for most questions on *P* values, but you should know more of the theory. *P* value is the probability of the result in question occurring, assuming that the distribution of occurrences used for the calculations is correct. Let's do a rough "for instance." Say you normally see 1 case of giardiasis in your office per week. Then one week you see 4 cases and you wonder if an epidemic of giardiasis has started. How often should you see 4 cases a week if you normally see only 1 case per week?

What you assume is chance variation results in a mean (average) incidence of giardiasis of 1 case per week and that the variation in occurrences is "per" a certain distribution. This is generally called the "null" or "chance" hypothesis. The distribution can be plotted from thousands of cases, or we can further assume it follows a standard distribution, such as the Poisson distribution. Assuming this is correct, what is the probability of 4 cases occurring in one week? What you do is go to a table that displays various values of the distribution and read the *P* value off the table. In this case, *P* = 0.019.

The way to read this: "Assuming that the average incidence of giardiasis is 1 case per week and further assuming that the weekly incidences of giardiasis fit into a normal Poisson distribution, then the probability of 4 cases per week occurring by chance is 1.9%." This seems small, and it is, but it does mean that you can expect to see 4 cases per week about once per year (if the assumptions are correct!). Now, if you see 4 cases again the following week ...!

Type 1 and Type 2 Errors

Type 1 = concluding that there is a difference (reject null hypothesis) when there is no difference. This is typically expressed by the *P* value. This reflects the willingness of the investigator to declare a benefit when there is none.

Type 2 = concluding that there is no difference (accept null hypothesis) when one exists. In other words, this is the likelihood that the trial will miss a true difference between the two test groups.

Meta-Analysis

Meta-analysis is the retrospective analysis of many studies concerned with the same topic. There are several methodological flaws and biases involved with meta-analyses, as well as several severe statistical restraints. Compiling studies with differing type 1 and type 2 errors is difficult. Other areas of difficulty include ages of participants and assumptions of the magnitude of differences expected among the experimental groups.

Confidence Interval Charts

Confidence interval (CI) charts are frequently used in meta-analyses—which are when results from all available relevant studies are analyzed together for greater statistical power.

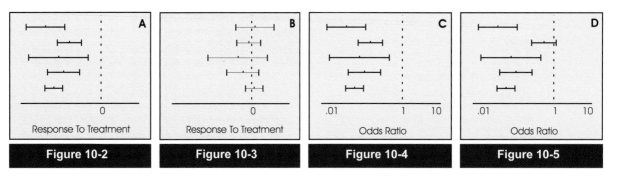

| Figure 10-2 | Figure 10-3 | Figure 10-4 | Figure 10-5 |

A CI of 95% is essentially the same as a $P < 0.05$. A CI of 99% is similar to $P < 0.01$.

Look at the charts (A–D) in Figure 10-2 through Figure 10-5. The vertical dotted line represents no effect—no response to treatment (A and B) or an odds ratio of 1 (C and D). In other representations, the vertical line may be given a specific number that represents the mean from the entire population or from controls. Each horizontal line on these charts represents the 95% confidence interval from one study.

If the "95% confidence interval" does not cross the vertical line, then the results are considered significant. For example, if you are reviewing a trial looking at response to treatment (i.e., vertical line = 0) and see that the 95% confidence interval is 0.5 to 1.9, you know the study shows a significant response. However, if the 95% confidence interval is –0.7 to 1.6, then it is a nonsignificant result!

Note that the charts depicted here could also be shown in a vertical format—with a horizontal dotted line representing the 0 or 1. Look at the chart sideways to see what this looks like!

Let's go over these charts so you can then tell at a glance how to interpret them:

• Chart A is a meta-analysis with each study showing a significant response to treatment.
• Chart B shows a similar meta-analysis in which not even one of the studies shows a significant response to treatment.
• Chart C shows a significantly different odds ratio in all studies reviewed. Odds ratio is a way of comparing whether the probability of an event is the same for 2 groups—usually comparing a control group and the study group (1 = same odds).
• Chart D shows 1 study with non-significant results but 4 others with significant results; therefore, the meta-analysis will show an overall significant result.

Number Needed to Treat

The number needed to treat (NNT) is the number of people who need to be treated for a period of time to prevent 1 event. NNT is calculated by taking the inverse of the absolute risk reduction between intervention and control groups.

Example: A new drug is studied to see if it can reduce heart failure mortality. Mortality in the treatment arm (active drug) was 10/100, while mortality in the placebo arm was 30/100 during a 4-year follow-up.

$$NNT = 1/(30/100 - 10/100) = 1/(0.3 - 0.1) = 1/0.2 = 5$$

This means 5 patients must be treated for 4 years to prevent 1 death.

Alternatively, NNH means number needed to harm. It is the number of patients who get a drug or intervention for each patient harmed.

OSTEOPOROSIS

OVERVIEW

Osteoporosis is decreased bone strength predisposing patients to bone fractures. Patients who get osteoporosis are postmenopausal females or both men and women with certain predisposing diseases, risk factors, and/or behaviors.

Osteoporosis is common in the elderly and generally suspected by clinical presentation (fragility fracture is a clinical diagnosis if postmenopausal). There are many risk factors for primary osteoporosis, but these have the highest known risk:

• History of fragility fracture in 1st degree relative
• Weight less than 127 lbs or BMI < 21
• Alcohol intake of 2 or more drinks/day
• Menopause before age 40
• Current or previous use of glucocorticoid therapy: > 3 months at a dose of > 5 mg/d of prednisone
• Cigarette smokers
• Personal history of fragility fracture

Patients with the following conditions should be screened regardless of age and gender:

• GI diseases (UC, Crohn's, celiac, gastric bypass, malabsorption)
• Endocrine disorders (hyperparathyroidism, Cushing syndrome, hypogonadism, hyperthyroidism)
• Medications (glucocorticoids, thyroxine over-replacement, lithium, phenobarbital, phenytoin, cyclosporine)

Quick Quiz

- What are the risk factors for osteoporosis?
- How do you screen for osteoporosis?
- How are the Z-score and T-score used in the evaluation of osteoporosis?
- Who should be treated for osteoporosis?
- What are the recommendations for all patients with osteoporosis?

- Rheumatoid arthritis, SLE
- Anorexia nervosa
- Prolonged bed rest or wheelchair bound

The most significant x-ray findings are multiple vertebral compression fractures (2/3 of vertebral fractures are painless).

The 3 most accurate methods of diagnosis (by determining loss of bone mineral density):

- Quantitative CT
- Dual photon absorptiometry (DPT)
- Dual energy x-ray absorptiometry (DEXA or DXA)

Quantitative CT scan gives a larger dose of radiation and is more expensive. CT scan and DPT take a lot of time. DXA is the preferred method. It is the quickest (about 15 minutes), the least expensive, and the most accurate! Precision of DXA is +/– 1–2%, whereas precision of DPT is +/– 2–5%.

Bone mineral density (BMD) reports usually have 2 results: the T-score and the Z-score. The T-score compares results with normal, young, healthy bone; a T-score of –1.0 means the BMD is 1 standard deviation (SD) less than normal—about 10% low. A T-score of –2.5 or lower is the definition of osteoporosis (about 25% below normal), whereas those between –1 and –2.5 suggest osteopenia. The Z-score compares the BMD result to age- and sex-matched controls and is now recommended for use in men and women younger than 50 years old. It is not used for treatment but rather to see if there is accelerated osteoporosis, which would suggest secondary factors—such as drugs—might be involved.

The National Osteoporosis Foundation, in collaboration with multiple organizations, implemented new guidelines in 2008 that recommend screening all women age 65 or older and all men 70 and older with DXA scans, and selectively screening women and men > 50 years if they have any osteoporosis risk factors, particularly those listed above.

The 2008 National Osteoporosis Foundation guidelines recommend that drug therapy should be considered in postmenopausal women and men > 50 years of age presenting with these findings:

- A hip or vertebral fracture
- T-score between –1.0 and –2.5 with other prior fractures (not hip or vertebral)
- T-score < –2.5 (remember this means a score like –3.0, –2.7 etc.; we are dealing with "less than" and negative numbers)
- T-score between –1.0 and –2.5 and secondary causes associated with high risk of fracture (steroid use or total immobilization)
- T-score between –1.0 and –2.5 and 10-year probability of hip fracture > 3% or a 10-year probability of any major osteoporosis-related fracture > 20% based on the U.S.-adapted WHO algorithm (these probabilities require calculations at www.shef.ac.uk/FRAX).

Universal recommendations for all patients (regardless of age or risk factors) with osteoporosis:

- Dietary calcium of 1,200–1,500 mg/day (include supplements if necessary, but higher amounts are not recommended due to increased risk of kidney stones and cardiovascular disease)
- Vitamin D intake of 800–1,000 IU of vitamin D_3 per day for adults > 50
- Regular weight-bearing exercise
- Fall prevention
- Avoid tobacco
- Avoid excess alcohol use (< 2 drinks/day)

DRUG THERAPY FOR OSTEOPOROSIS

All drugs that increase bone density do so by affecting bone remodeling. They can either increase the buildup (stimulate osteoblasts) or decrease breakdown (inhibit osteoclasts). A categorization of the drugs, which is based on these effects on bone remodeling, is anabolic vs. anticatabolic. Anabolic agents stimulate both osteoblasts and osteoclasts but stimulate the osteoblasts more, leading to a net increase in bone building and increased bone density. Anticatabolic agents inhibit osteoclasts, thereby decreasing the resorptive process:

Anabolic agents (stimulate osteoblasts): Parathyroid hormone (teriparatide) is currently the only one available. Teriparatide can be used for only 2 years (because of cumulative increased risk of osteosarcoma) and, once discontinued, patients need to use a bisphosphonate.

Anticatabolic agents (antiresorptive: inhibits osteoclasts) includes the rest of the osteoporosis drugs:

- HRT (hormone replacement therapy)
- Bisphosphonates
  - Oral bisphosphonates: alendronate (Fosamax®), ibandronate (Boniva®, also available in IV form, see next), risedronate (Actonel®)
  - Injectable bisphosphonates: ibandronate and zoledronate (Reclast®)

- Calcitonin salmon
- Raloxifene (Evista®)

A few notes on these drugs:

Teriparatide is the only anabolic agent currently available. Parathyroid hormone causes both an increase in bone buildup and an increase in bone resorption—but the net effect is to build more bone than it breaks down.

HRT may prevent or reverse the development of osteoporosis, but its use in the peri- and postmenopausal woman is a two-edged sword. Most recommend not using HRT as 1ˢᵗ-line therapy! See HRT on page 10-13.

Bisphosphonates are analogs of pyrophosphate and, like estrogen and other anticatabolic agents, inhibit bone resorption. Bisphosphonates and HRT appear to have an additive effect. They effectively act as antagonists of parathyroid hormone, which causes resorption—a release of calcium from the bone into the serum.

Bisphosphonates, especially IV, have been associated with osteonecrosis of the jaw. Use caution if using these drugs in patients who will be having extensive dental surgery. Another very important side effect is severe muscle/joint/bone pain. Odd fractures of the long bones (femur) have been reported in patients receiving bisphosphonates.

- Alendronate is an option when a patient is uncomfortable with HRT or HRT is contraindicated. Alendronate is both poorly absorbed and a rare cause of severe esophagitis (although this is less of a problem with weekly dosing); the patient must carefully follow the recommendations to take it with a full glass of water on an empty stomach and not eat or lie down for 30 minutes after ingestion.
- Risedronate was FDA-approved in April 2000 for the prevention and treatment of postmenopausal osteoporosis. It has the same clinical effect as alendronate but may have fewer GI side effects. Even so, take the same dosing precautions as with alendronate.
- Ibandronate is the first once-monthly medication approved for postmenopausal osteoporosis.

Calcitonin salmon nasal spray at 200 mg/d increases bone mineral density and decreases risk of vertebral fractures. There is no evidence that it decreases hip fracture risk.

Raloxifene. During the development of antiestrogens, it was discovered that some substances that block the effect of estrogen on some tissues actually mimic estrogen on others! These are called selective estrogen receptor modulators (SERMs). Examples are tamoxifen and raloxifene. The effect of raloxifene on bone and lipid levels is similar to, but less than, estrogen—however, it exerts estrogen-antagonistic effects on the breast and uterus and may be less likely to cause cancer than traditional HRT. Raloxifene is FDA-approved for both prevention and treatment of postmenopausal osteoporosis.

Fractures are the most serious consequence of osteoporosis. There are 1.5 million fractures per year due to osteoporosis, with 300,000 of those due to hip fracture. Mortality due to hip fractures is about 20% within the first year! Femoral neck and intratrochanteric fractures account for 97% of hip fractures.

Femoral neck fractures are intracapsular and occur below the femoral head but above the trochanters. Displaced femoral neck fractures often disrupt the blood supply to the femoral head and result in osteonecrosis and/or nonunion; therefore, the treatment of choice is either femoral head replacement or total hip arthroplasty. Nondisplaced femoral neck fractures have a low incidence of osteonecrosis and nonunion, so these are usually treated with internal fixation using pins or screws.

Intertrochanteric fractures are extracapsular and are usually treated with internal fixation with a "sliding hip screw."

In both types of fracture, the main goal is to achieve mobility and function as soon as possible, thereby avoiding the morbidity and spiraling complications due to poor mobility.

Deep vein thrombosis (DVT) occurs in 48% of hip fracture patients without anticoagulants. With anticoagulation, DVT occurs in 24% and 27%, respectively, for those on warfarin or subQ low-molecular-weight heparin.

Other complications of hip fractures are pressure ulcers, constipation, and fecal impaction.

GERIATRICS

DEMOGRAPHICS

Life expectancy correlates with race and gender. Caucasian women live the longest; in a tie for 2ⁿᵈ place are African-American women and Caucasian men. African-American men have the shortest life spans. Generally, women live longer than men, are less likely to remarry, lack money to take care of all their needs, and are more often disabled as they age.

60–84% of patients > 65 years old will have hypertension, and roughly 20% have diabetes. Cancer is now the leading cause of death in adults younger than 85 years (followed by heart disease and stroke). Many studies show that elderly patients are not offered the same life-saving procedures as younger patients with the same disease states, even though age has no adverse effect on outcomes of the interventions. Know that age alone is not enough of a reason to withhold an intervention.

If a patient lives to be 75 years old, he will most likely live to age 86. And those who live to 85 years are likely to live to age 91.

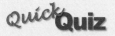

Quick Quiz

- A patient on alendronate presents with difficulty swallowing. What is the likely etiology?
- What is the most serious consequence of osteoporosis?
- How do you diagnose "frailty?"
- What assessments should be done periodically in elderly patients?
- What are the major features of delirium, using the Confusion Assessment Method?

"Frailty" affects a large number of elderly patients. It can be caused by comorbid illnesses and/or disability but not necessarily so. Frail patients are more likely to fall, become disabled, or die. Make a diagnosis of "frailty" if ≥ 3 of the following are present:

- Unintentional loss of ≥ 10 lbs/1 year
- Exhaustion due to lack of endurance
- Decreased hand strength
- Walking slowly
- Reduced activity

ASSESSMENT

All geriatric patients should have a specific interval assessment of "function" because functionality is related to longevity. Functional assessment evaluates several components:

- Activities of daily living (ADLs)
- Instrumental activities of daily living (IADLs)
- Cognition
- Hearing
- Vision
- Gait and balance
- Nutrition (discussed separately)
- Driving ability

Start by assessing ADLs: Can the patient dress, bathe, feed, use the bathroom, and move around without help? IADLs are those activities that connect the patient with the community: Can she manage her money, take her own medication, manage transportation, make phone calls, do the shopping and housework, and make her meals?

Assessment of cognition looks for evidence of dementia and delirium.

Assessing dementia: A quick way is to use the Mini-Mental Status exam (MMSE) or the Mini-Cog (easier to remember) to assess dementia. To perform the Mini-Cog, ask the patient to remember 3 words, and then ask him to draw a clock showing a specific time. After he's drawn the clock, ask him to recite the 3 words. Score by giving 1 point for each word remembered correctly and 2 points for an accurate clock (0–2 = dementia).

Assessing delirium: The best tool to assess delirium is the Confusion Assessment Method (CAM; 94–100% sensitive; 90–95% specific). See Table 10-7. Delirium is present when patients have features 1 and 2 with either 3 or 4.

More on dementia and delirium on page 10-14.

Hearing and vision can be assessed using traditional instruments such as the whisper test and the Snellen eye chart. The whisper test is performed by covering the ear that is not being tested, then whispering a question while standing about 2 feet away. If the patient responds correctly, then no more testing is required. Give the patient 6 tries. Refer for further audiometric testing if the patient answers 3 or more questions (out of 6) incorrectly.

Gait and balance are assessed well with the timed Get-Up-and-Go test. Have the patient get up from a chair and walk 10 feet, then turn around and come back to sit. If it takes him longer than 20 seconds, then he is at high risk for falls; 10–20 seconds puts him at moderate risk. More specifics below about falls in Mobility and Gait.

Know that elderly (and teens) have more driving violations compared to the general population. Usually, patient performance on the vision, hearing, and gait assessment will give you an adequate assessment of a patient's ability to operate a vehicle. Formal assessment is offered for the elderly through departments of motor vehicles.

NUTRITION

We become less active as we age, and we lose muscle and body fat (more muscle than fat). Nutritional

Table 10-7: Delirium Assessment Tool—Confusion Assessment Method	
Feature 1	Acute onset and fluctuating course: Is mental status acutely changed from baseline, and does the change fluctuate throughout the day?
Feature 2	Inattention: Is there a problem focusing attention (e.g., easily distracted)?
Feature 3	Disorganized thinking: Is conversation rambling or irrelevant? Are ideas illogical in flow?
Feature 4	Altered level of consciousness: Is the patient alert (normal state), hyper-alert, drowsy but easily aroused, difficult to arouse, or unarousable?

requirements are reduced, so generally, older people eat less. Malnutrition is still an issue for them, though, because of declining abilities and comorbid systemic disease.

Malnutrition is diagnosed in any of the following circumstances:

• Unintentional weight loss of ≥ 10 lbs/6 months
• BMI < 22
• Albumin < 3.8 g/dL
• Cholesterol < 160 mg/dL
• Any vitamin deficiency

When malnutrition is diagnosed, thoroughly assess for modifiable risks; e.g., decreased access to nutritious food, denture or teeth problems, untreated medical illness, inability to perform IADLs such as grocery shopping.

The declining appetite and energy needs with aging are associated with a natural replacement of carbohydrates for fats. Counsel geriatric patients to increase their daily fluid and fiber intake and to eat healthy fats (monounsaturated and omega-3s) such as olive oil, nuts, avocados, and fish. Vitamin supplements are useful in patients who are poor eaters because this age group is especially vulnerable to deficiencies of vitamin D, B_{12}, and calcium.

The National Institute on Alcohol Abuse and Alcoholism and the American Geriatrics Society have recommendations on healthy alcohol intake for people older than 65 years—no more than 2–3 drinks/day and/or 7 drinks/week, with lower amounts for people taking meds with side effects that are potentiated by alcohol.

MOBILITY AND GAIT

Falling

Age is associated with increased instability and falls. 50% of patients age 80 and older fall each year! The elderly have a stiffer, less agile gait with decreased position reflexes. 5% of falls result in fractures and, if the patient cannot get up, possibly hypothermia and dehydration.

Aging is associated with decreased proprioception and baroreceptor reflexes, so orthostatic hypotension and swaying is common. There is also an increased incidence of postprandial falls in the elderly—probably due to hypotension from ingestion of carbohydrates.

The major predictor for fracture from a fall is osteoporosis.

Risk factors for falls:

• Age
• Female gender
• Past history of falls
• Rugs, untidiness, and dim lighting in the home
• Poor vision
• Orthostatic hypotension
• Unsteady gait

• Cognitive impairment
• Musculoskeletal disease
• Cardiovascular disease (e.g., syncope)
• Psychotropic drug use

The drugs most commonly implicated are benzodiazepines, antidepressants, neuroleptic agents, and blood pressure medications. Know that using forms of physical restraint increases the risk of serious falls and injuries, so avoid physical restraints when possible.

There are 5 quick office tests that can be done to assess the risk for fall in the elderly:

1) Timed Get-Up-and-Go test (see Assessment on page 10-9)
2) Gait speed (slower = ↑ risk)
3) Tandem (heel-to-toe) walk
4) Visual acuity
5) Calf circumference (smaller = ↑ risk)

Workup for the patient with falls includes a good history and physical exam, with emphasis on a multidisciplinary assessment and evaluation for a cardiovascular cause. Do a syncope workup if the patient does not remember the fall or if the history is suggestive. Also think about weakness associated with osteomalacia as a cause—especially in nursing home patients who are bedridden and never get in the sunshine. Check $25\text{-}(OH)_2\text{-}D$ if you suspect osteomalacia, and treat deficiency if found because treatment decreases fall risk.

Anticipatory guidance for falls may include restriction of certain activities, improving the lighting at home (use night lights), decreasing hazards (remove rugs and loose carpets), and placing extra supports (bars in the shower). Exercise (especially focused on balance and resistance training) is very important in helping patients maintain mobility and strength, reduce falls, and prolong survival.

Immobility

Patients adapt to bedrest; and the longer a patient is immobilized, the harder it is to ambulate again. Immobilization causes decreased ADH secretion → diuresis → decreased blood volume → orthostatic symptoms. Also, immobilization causes muscle atrophy. The heart continually deconditions after 2 days of bedrest. The elderly are more affected by bedrest because they have less reserve than young people. Treat with rehabilitation.

Know that prolonged immobility is associated with development of hypercalcemia (although this is more common in teens and young adults after traumatic immobilization). The hypercalcemia improves with mobilization.

Decubitus Ulcers

Sustained pressure over a prominent bone is the main etiologic factor. Shearing and friction tear the skin and cause necrosis with ulceration. Moist environments (notably, urinary incontinence) increase the risk. Know

- What are the criteria that diagnose malnutrition?
- Which factors, associated with aging, predispose patients to imbalance and falls?
- What are risk factors for falls in the elderly?
- How does immobilization affect serum calcium levels?
- What factors are associated with development of decubitus ulcers?
- What is the role of wet-to-dry dressings in decubitus ulcer treatment?

that decubiti in nursing home patients increase their mortality (usually from osteomyelitis and bacteremia/sepsis). Also know that malnutrition (≥ 10 lb weight loss in past 6 months) increases the risk for development of ulcers.

There are 4 stages of decubitus ulcerations.

- Stage I is non-blanching erythema (reddish macules).
- Stage II is partial-thickness skin loss (small superficial ulcer).
- Stage III is full-thickness skin loss.
- Stage IV is loss of tissue down to the muscle, tendon, or bone.

Most common places that pressure ulcers occur are the heels, trochanter, sacrum, and iliac crest.

Bed-bound patients should be rotated from side to side (30-degree angle) every 2 hours. This prevents contact against bony prominences mentioned above. Special mattresses and heel/elbow pads also help, but it's controversial whether most interventions actually prevent ulcers.

In established ulcers, keep pressure off the area; and if an eschar exists, remove it for proper staging. The workup then includes determining whether any arterial or venous insufficiency exists and treating any infection or maintaining a "clean" ulcer.

Infected ulcers require debridement of necrotic tissue back to healthy granulation tissue, using either "chemical" topical treatments or a scalpel.

Next, the wound has to be cleaned and dressed properly. Know that saline cleansing is best because it is gentle on growing tissue, and that iodines or peroxides kill tissue if used repeatedly. The choices for wound dressings are wide and variable. Follow the advice given by the wound care physical therapist. Know wet-to-dry dressings as a means for debriding wounds have fallen out of favor because they too often damage friable new tissue.

Give antibiotics, in addition to local wound care, if the patient is systemically ill. Use deep wound cultures to guide your choice.

Wounds will not heal in malnourished patients, so strictly follow the recommendations of the nutritionists to provide adequate increased nutrition.

Know that wounds that develop in the setting of arterial or venous insufficiency will not heal unless the local blood flow is corrected—most often via surgical intervention. Sometimes this is feasible, sometimes not, depending on the patient's comorbidities.

Stage 1 and 2 ulcers heal quickly, but stages 3 and 4 usually take months.

IMMUNITY

Decreased immunity is age-related. Total T- and B-cell numbers stay the same, but the number of CD4 T cells increases with age, while the number of CD8 T cells decreases with age. Also, only half of the T cells remain competent, which is why herpes zoster and reactivation tuberculosis is often seen in the elderly.

PHARMACOLOGY

The elderly are very sensitive to drugs for the following reasons:

- Pharmacokinetics change with aging (changes in absorption and metabolism), which leads to increased concentrations of drugs.
- The volume of distribution for a drug increases because of the proportional increase of body fat compared to muscle.
- Excretion decreases, consistent with age-related decreases in renal and hepatic function.
- Pharmacodynamics of aging → increased effects of drugs, especially opioids and benzodiazepines.

General rules for medications in the elderly:

- Start meds at a low dose—usually about 1/2 the dose required for the general population and gradually titrate up to the normal therapeutic dose. If the patient gets into trouble at the therapeutic dose, try reducing the dose gradually—many elderly patients get satisfactory responses with subtherapeutic doses.
- Any adverse event should be assumed to be drug-related until proven otherwise.
- Always look to see if a prescribed drug is the cause of new symptoms before prescribing a new drug to symptomatically treat the new symptoms.
- Look at an elderly patient's medicine record for prescription of an atypical antipsychotic (see Delirium on page 10-14) if he is institutionalized and falling. These are the most common causes of falls in nursing homes.
- Errors in self-administration increase dramatically once a patient is prescribed 3 or more medications. Elderly patients get very confused with pills that look alike and between generic and brand names.

Many elderly patients are dependent on low-dose benzodiazepines (BDZs) or narcotics. For these patients, you should attempt a slow withdrawal of these medications. These have often been misprescribed as treatment for anxiety, insomnia, depression, chronic pain, and drug withdrawal. Slowly taper following these general principles: Taper BDZs over 3–6 months after switching to an equivalent dosage of a water-soluble BDZ, such as oxazepam (slower onset, less addictive potential). With narcotic dependence, first determine the cause of pain (if any) and treat it with a non-narcotic drug (NSAID, acetaminophen). Avoid long half-life narcotics in treating geriatric pain.

Know that up to 75% of the elderly population in some studies use herbal supplements. Many do not divulge this information unless you ask directly.

ENDOCRINE

The only specific hormonal change that occurs with aging is ovarian failure: the average age of menopause is 51 years. The hypothalamic-pituitary-gonadal axis is also disturbed in men, but not as predictably as in women. In both sexes, the adrenal zona glomerulosa declines in synthesis of DHEA and the pituitary secretion of growth hormone wanes (and subsequently, also levels of IGF-1). Many other hormones are normal in the amount produced but do not function as well.

Many of these hormone perturbations are felt to be associated with the aging process, but none are conclusively linked. Growth hormone reduction appears to be associated with loss of muscle mass and strength. But supplementation is not encouraged because it is associated with too many side effects.

The pineal gland does not produce melatonin normally, and this may cause poor sleep and insomnia. Some patients are helped with melatonin supplementation.

Aging patients have a reduction in the clearance of thyroid hormone, so replacement hormone for hypothyroidism can be started at a lower dose. TSH increases with age, especially in women (see the Endocrinology section); but at this time, a rising TSH without an accompanied decrease in T4 does not merit treatment for hypothyroidism.

Testosterone production decreases in men with age, but the effect is variable. However, the rate of sperm production is stable from ages 20 to 70 years! FSH and LH also decline but disproportionately compared to the more drastic decline in testosterone. The low testosterone production is most likely due to declining testicular function and not to hypothalamic disease.

Low testosterone is believed to be related to the following, although direct causation has not been proven:

• Decreased sexual function
• Decreased bone mineral density
• Decreased muscle mass (and increased fat)
• Decreased muscle strength
• Decreased mentation

The collection of the above, in association with reduced free testosterone, is called "andropause." The Endocrine Society has guidelines (2006) for treatment of certain males with andropause who have symptoms and a serum testosterone < 200 ng/dL, with a treatment goal of 300–400 ng/dL. In spite of this recommendation, there are no good studies that prove a treatment benefit. Do not screen elderly men and do not treat men with low levels if they do not have symptoms.

Vitamin D deficiency is common because of decreased intake, decreased absorption, reduced sun exposure, and poor conversion of the storage to active form of vitamin D. Vitamin D intake in patients older than 70 years should be at least 600 IU/day, and many patients probably should be getting supplements. Decreased calcium intake is also common. 1,500 mg of elemental Ca/day is recommended in patients 65 and older.

Bone

Osteoporosis

The majority of women over 80 years old have osteoporosis. According to current guidelines (see Osteoporosis on page 10-6), women 65 years of age and older should be screened with the DXA scan at least once. If the patient has any risk factors for vitamin D deficiency (especially poor diet or lack of sun exposure), check stores by measuring $25\text{-}(OH)_2\text{-}D$.

Paget Disease

Paget disease of bone occurs in about 1% of people > 40 years old in the U.S. It is usually diagnosed after discovering an isolated elevation of alkaline phosphatase in an asymptomatic person. The disease results from a mismatch of osteoclast and osteoblast activity (remodeling), causing changes seen on x-ray, bone scan, CT, or MRI in localized areas. The bones are more brittle, vascular, and larger—leading to arthritis, high-output heart failure, and nerve compression, respectively

Etiology: Viral trigger in a host with certain genes.

Diagnosis is strongly suggested by bone scan results. Patients with Paget disease have focal areas of marked increased uptake.

Treatment is not required in the majority of patients and is not curative but may be needed if heart failure, bone pain, nerve compression, or hearing loss develops.

Drugs used: Bisphosphonates (etidronate, pamidronate, and alendronate) given orally or IV are effective in the treatment of Paget disease. SC or IM calcitonin has also been shown to be effective.

GENERAL INTERNAL MEDICINE

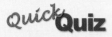

Diabetes

Aging is associated with decreased carbohydrate tolerance, shown as a slight increase in fasting glucose. And now we know that insulin sensitivity and production declines with age. Elderly patients with diabetes get the same micro- and macrovascular complications as younger patients, but the elderly have to be specifically watched for life-threatening hypoglycemia, hypotension, and drug-drug interactions.

Hypoglycemia more often presents as cognitive impairment in the elderly, rather than tremulousness and sweats. Most likely causes of hypoglycemia are insulins and the insulin secretagogues (sulfonylureas and meglitinides), especially the 1st generation (chlorpropamide). Glyburide has about twice the incidence of hypoglycemia in the elderly compared to glipizide (27% vs. 14%!) and is no longer recommended for use as a 1st-line sulfonylurea by the American Diabetes Association (ADA).

Be cautious with metformin use in the elderly because of the high prevalence of renal insufficiency in this population and the tendency of these patients to develop lactic acidosis. Measure CrCl prior to use of metformin in patients > age 80, and do not give the drug to any patient with a CrCl < 60, regardless of age.

Rosiglitazone is no longer recommended for use by the ADA. Pioglitazone also should be avoided in the elderly, due to the risk of edema and precipitation of CHF. The jury is still out, also, on whether these drugs are associated with an increased risk of cardiac events and stroke.

Remember to adjust downward the insulin doses as renal function declines with age, especially as GFR drops below 50 cc/min.

Hyperthyroidism

People > 60 years old with thyroid disease are more likely to have vague symptoms that could indicate either hyper- or hypothyroidism. Features of classic hyperthyroidism, such as hyperreflexia, heat intolerance, tremor, nervousness, polydipsia, and increased appetite, are usually absent in elderly persons. "Apathetic hyperthyroidism" can be seen in elderly patients and presents as apathy, fatigue, anorexia/weight loss, and tachycardia. Atrial fibrillation and anorexia can occur in older patients with hypothyroidism; we rarely see these symptoms in hypothyroid younger patients.

Hormone Replacement Therapy (HRT)

Estrogen replacement is the best option for alleviating vasomotor and other menopausal symptoms and can be used safely for short periods.

The most substantial data we have on HRT are from the Women's Health Initiative (WHI), published in 2002. Prior to this study, the standard of care (based on observational data) had been to prescribe HRT to postmenopausal women to protect their bones and prevent coronary disease. The WHI data, however, showed that HRT (estrogen only) is ineffective long term for preventing heart disease, and that combination HRT is associated with a slight increased risk for heart disease, stroke, venous thrombosis, and breast cancer. Both groups had an increased incidence of gall bladder disease. Combined therapy did reduce the risks of colon cancer and osteoporotic fractures, but not enough to justify these increased risks.

Follow-up analysis of the WHI data tells us that the women who experienced the heart disease and strokes were the older women in the study.

Conclusions from WHI that drive practice today:

- Combination HRT is associated with an increase in heart disease, stroke, venous clotting, breast cancer, and gall bladder disease. Unopposed estrogen use was not associated with the heart disease or breast cancer risks.
- Younger, perimenopausal women do not appear to have an increased risk for heart disease and stroke with combination HRT. But older women do.
- Estrogen alone causes endometrial hyperplasia and increases risk of endometrial cancer. Combination estrogen-progestin in women with a uterus is not associated with this risk.
- Premature ovarian failure (menopause before age 40) can be safely treated with combination HRT until the woman is 50 years old, then stop and discuss the risks.

The important concept: Do not give women > 50 years old combination HRT because it increases their risks for stroke, heart disease, breast cancer, venous clotting, and gallstones—and the reduction in fractures is inadequate to compensate for these increased risks. Perimenopausal use of estrogen replacement is discussed later in Office Gynecology (see page 10-53).

NEUROLOGIC

Delirium

Delirium is confusion with altered consciousness. It is a common problem in the elderly. Main features are abnormal attention span (easily distracted), disorganized thinking (may have hallucinations), and altered consciousness (with increased or decreased mental activity) that fluctuates during the day and typically worsens at night. Patients with underlying dementia and/or stroke are at highest risk.

Common precipitating causes include drugs, poor nutritional status, acute illness (e.g., infections, volume depletion). Know that physical restraints and bladder catheters can incite delirium as well. In the post-op period, uncontrolled pain is a major cause, especially in geriatric patients with hip fractures.

1/3 of cases will be caused by drugs. Drugs to be aware of especially include meperidine, NSAIDs, any new antimicrobial, diphenhydramine, all cardiovascular drugs and antidepressants, antiemetics, baclofen, H_2 receptor blockers, sleep-inducers, and herbals (e.g., St. John's Wort and valerian root). Acute discontinuation of alcohol, benzodiazepines (BDZs), SSRIs, and pain medications may cause withdrawal delirium.

Know that in the elderly, delirium may be the only manifestation of illness. Any patient who becomes delirious should be thoroughly evaluated for a serious precipitating cause.

Evaluate the confused patient with an objective tool such as the MMSE or the CAM (see page 10-9). Physical exam should focus on identifying an underlying acute illness that may be associated with confusion (e.g., drug abuse, hepatic failure, uremia, head injuries, stroke, and seizures). Work up the central nervous system (imaging and LP) if no cause is found after a thorough search.

Differentiate delirium from "sundowning": Sundowning is a disturbance in behavior that occurs predictably in the evening among some patients who live in chronic care environments. It is not associated with a precipitating illness and is not delirium. With sundowning, usually the care facility can tell you that the patient predictably deteriorates at night.

Treatment of delirium is supportive with focus on diagnosis and treatment of the underlying cause. Calendars and orienting signs, nightlights, newspapers, a radio, glasses, and hearing aids help stabilize and prevent decompensation. It is also necessary to minimize daily stress.

Pharmacologic treatment of delirium in the elderly is tough because the meds themselves can worsen the confusion. Low-dose haloperidol is still recommended for most patients, but watch for prolongation of the QT interval—and do not use it in patients with Parkinson's. Alternative drugs include the atypical antipsychotics: risperidone, olanzapine (Zyprexa®), and quetiapine (Seroquel®). These drugs are as effective with fewer side effects than full-dose haloperidol, but they are expensive. Don't use BDZs in delirious patients because they make patients more confused and drowsy.

Use of a "sitter" and other nonpharmacologic interventions are the best first choices in both "real life" and on the Board exam. Remember to avoid physical restraint of geriatric patients at all costs because it precipitates delirium and causes falls.

Dementia

Patients with dementia have a progressive deterioration of cognition that is insidious and chronic—but without altered consciousness, as with delirium. The deterioration can be either very gradual or step-wise (related to the underlying cause). The cognitive impairment presents as:

- Difficulty learning and remembering new information
- Decreased problem-solving of both simple and complex tasks
- Decline in spatial organization → they get lost
- Trouble with impulse control → unusual behavior

Some decline in cognition occurs with normal aging, but memory loss is mild and should not affect the patient's daily living or be especially noticeable by family.

Most patients in the U.S. with dementia are diagnosed with Alzheimer disease (80%), followed by multi-infarct dementia. Lewy body dementia and dementia from Parkinson's are less common syndromes. See the Neurology section for a more thorough discussion.

Depression can look like dementia, especially in the elderly. A couple of ways to tell the difference: Depressed patients often present complaining of memory loss, while demented patients are brought in by family or friends. Depressed patients have a depressed affect and slowing with completion of the MMSE or mini-cog, while demented patients have a more normal affect and try hard. Assessment tools can help identify the true cognitive defects of dementia (see page 10-9). A score of < 24 points on the MMSE is consistent with dementia/delirium.

At this time, the position of the U.S. Preventive Services Task Force on screening for dementia is that there is insufficient evidence to recommend for or against it.

First-line treatment for Alzheimer's is the cholinesterase inhibitors (CIs): Donepezil (Aricept®), tacrine (Cognex®), rivastigmine (Exelon®), and galantamine (Razadyne®). Tacrine is associated with liver toxicity. Best results with CIs are achieved in mild-moderate Alzheimer dementia, but other causes of dementia (e.g., multi-infarct and Lewy bodies) sometimes also improve. CIs do not help patients with Huntington disease, however. CIs can be combined with memantine (Namenda®), which is an N-methyl-d-aspartate receptor antagonist.

CIs provide a small benefit and help some patients carry out their activities of daily living (ADLs). Data are

Quick Quiz

- What are the main features of delirium? Precipitating factors?
- How is delirium different from "sundowning?"
- What is the recommended drug for elderly patients with delirium?
- How is dementia different from delirium?
- What are the 2 most common causes of dementia in the U.S.?
- When do patients derive the greatest benefit from Alzheimer treatment?
- What are common symptoms of geriatric depression? Side effects of meds?
- Name some medications typically associated with insomnia in the elderly.

conflicting on their long-term effects. Not every patient receives benefit, either. The combination of cholinesterase inhibitor plus memantine appears to be better than CI alone.

Vitamin E is no longer recommended as a supplement because it may increase the risk of heart disease and death. Ginkgo biloba extract and vitamins A and D have not been shown in clinical trials to improve cognition in elderly patients.

In March 2008, the ACP published dementia treatment guidelines. These guidelines were evidence-based and demonstrated little benefit for any of the current cholinesterase inhibitors or memantine; the authors recommended that individual patient factors would likely determine need to initiate therapy because the data were not very compelling for initiating therapy in any patient. Know that the benefit from treating Alzheimer's is greatest early in the disease, and the cholinesterase inhibitors should be stopped in patients with severe dementia.

Depression

Depression is the most common mental problem in the elderly. It is particularly likely to occur in those who live in institutionalized settings and/or have chronic diseases, especially just after a severe sickness or in states of chronic pain. Know that the depressed elderly (especially men) make up 1/4 of the successful suicide attempts in the U.S.

Look for dysphoria, psychomotor slowing, anorexia, weight loss, and multiple "aches and pains." Know that insomnia is associated with depression, especially in the elderly, although it is not known whether it is a symptom or a cause. Depression-associated delusions are more common in the elderly than in the general population. Pay special attention to the elderly man with depressed mood, hopelessness, chronic pain, and insomnia because his suicide risk is particularly high.

A host of substances and drugs can potentiate depression, including alcohol, BDZs, opiates, and barbiturates. Untreated thyroid disease, diabetes, and pain are organic causes.

Treatment is usually psychotherapy combined with antidepressants +/– electroconvulsive therapy (ECT). Exercise helps too. Selective serotonin reuptake inhibitors (SSRIs) are the 1st-line drugs because they have fewer side effects than other choices. The most common reason for stopping these agents is sexual dysfunction! (See Table 10-8.)

With antidepressants in the elderly, always start with low doses (typically 1/2 the normal dose) and increase slowly with the goal of eventually reaching the normal therapeutic dose. See patients (or call them) within 2 weeks after initiating meds. Watch for the side effects of hyponatremia and tremor in elderly patients on SSRIs. It takes about 8 weeks to see improvement. 6–12 months is the usual duration of treatment. Know that treating a patient's depression can help their comorbidities improve as well.

Sleep Disturbance

Insomnia

Sleep disturbance is a common problem in elderly persons, and normal aging is associated with more frequent awakenings. These disturbances include difficulty falling asleep (> 30 minutes), frequent awakenings, waking too early, and feeling generally unrestored. When the disturbance also causes problems for the patient during the day (e.g., poor concentration, moodiness, sleepiness, fatigue), it is classified as "insomnia."

Know what is not insomnia:

- Some people can sleep well for only a few hours and have no problem functioning the next day. These patients simply have short-duration sleep.
- People who have not slept voluntarily (because of work or whatever) and can easily fall asleep during the day are classified as having "insufficient sleep" or "sleep deprivation," not insomnia.

Insomnia, especially in the elderly, is associated with worsening of hypertension, heart disease, lung disease, urinary incontinence, chronic pain, and depression.

History should focus on characterizing the sleep disturbance (sleep logs help) and identifying any untreated comorbidities and/or precipitants (e.g., naps, stress, newly stopped or started meds, alcohol, caffeine, nicotine).

Medications specifically associated with insomnia include corticosteroids, beta-blockers, beta-agonists, and stopping sedatives or pain meds.

Labs are recommended only to diagnose potential comorbidities (e.g., hyperthyroidism, restless legs). Sleep studies are unnecessary until a patient has failed to respond to conservative management.

Treatment should be directed at improving any poorly managed comorbidities, and advise the patient on good sleep hygiene:

- Set a schedule for sleep and stick to it.
- Get in the bed only when you're sleepy. When you're rested, get up.
- Minimize excess light and sound in the bedroom.
- Exercise during the day and at least 4 hours before bedtime.
- Stay away from caffeine, nicotine, and alcohol near bedtime.

- Eat dinner or an evening snack to prevent bedtime hunger.
- Don't fight sleep. If you can't sleep for > 20 minutes, get up and do something relaxing (reading or music). No bright lights or TV.

The most efficacious treatment in patients with uncomplicated insomnia is behavioral—not pharmacologic. Elderly patients are especially susceptible to bad outcomes from sleep drugs.

Benzodiazepines actually do help by decreasing the

Table 10-8: Antidepressants, Selective Receptor Blockers

Drug	T 1/2 (hrs)	Mechanism of Action/Blocks ...	Notes	Drug of Choice for ...	Caution (!) in patients ...
Fluoxetine (Prozac®, Serafem®)*	72	SSRI	May cause anxiety and insomnia		... with insomnia
Paroxetine (Paxil®, Pexeva®)*	20	SSRI	Most anticholinergic of the SSRIs Sedating in some		... in whom anticholinergics are to be avoided. ... with insomnia
Sertraline (Zoloft®)*	25	SSRI	GI discomfort is common		... with insomnia ... with irritable bowel
Fluvoxamine (Luvox®)*	15	SSRI	Most sedating of the SSRIs	... pts with agitation ... pts with insomnia ... pts with obsessive-compulsive disorder	... with irritable bowel
Citalopram (Celexa®)*	35	SSRI	May cause anxiety and insomnia, N/V, headache		
Nefazodone (Serzone®)	3***	SSRI and 5-HT2 and has anti-alpha adrenergic activity	Maintains sleep architecture Sexual dysfunction is unlikely	... pts with insomnia; ... to maintain sexual activity	... on benzodiazepines or antihistamines (interacts with cytochrome P-450 system)**
Venlafaxine (Effexor®)	4	SSRI and norepinephrine reuptake and some dopamine reuptake			... with insomnia ... with HTN—usually increases blood pressure, so not used in these patients
Bupropion (Wellbutrin®)	15	Reuptake of dopamine and some norepinephrine	Sedation is unlikely Sexual dysfunction is unlikely		... with insomnia ... with HTN—may increase blood pressure
Mirtazapine (Remeron®)	20	Presynaptic alpha2 receptor (increases seritonin and norepi release) AND 5-HT2 AND 5-HT3	Agitation is unlikely Sexual dysfunction is unlikely Good for insomniacs	... pts with insomnia; ... to maintain sexual activity	Most anticholinergic of all these ... with HTN—may increase blood pressure

*All the SSRIs have a tendency to cause agitation, sedation, and sexual dysfunction. Pure SSRIs are not likely to increase blood pressure.
**May use loratadine (Claritin®) or lorazepam (Ativan®) with nefazodone.
***T 1/2 is higher than this in elderly, especially women.
Note 1: Buspirone is a 5-HT1A agonist that can be combined with an SSRI to decrease the dose or improve efficacy.
Note 2: Any SSRI may cause an increase of suicidal thought or actions in 1 of 50 age < 18 years.

Quick Quiz

- What is the role of benzodiazepines in treatment of insomnia?
- What dangerous side effects are sometimes seen with both benzodiazepine and non-benzodiazepine sleep agents?
- What is a common condition associated with restless leg syndrome?

frequency of awakenings, reducing time to fall asleep, and increasing duration of sleep. But they have many negative side effects, including addiction, loss of memory, and accumulation of metabolites.

Non-benzodiazepine insomnia drugs, such as zolpidem (Ambien®), zaleplon (Sonata®), and eszopiclone (Lunesta®), have more selective effects than BDZs because they affect only a portion of the receptor subunits that DBZ's affect. Because of this, non-BDZs tend to have more sedative than anxiolytic effects than BDZs. Additionally, they don't have as many side effects as BDZs.

Even so, both BDZs and non-BDZs can cause confusion, wandering, imbalance, and daytime grogginess in the elderly—hence both classes are avoided in geriatric patients.

Many sleep-aid drugs in both the BDZ and non-BDZ classes have received FDA-required label changes, indicating that the drugs can cause an hypnotic state that allows patients to attempt complex tasks while sleeping → bizarre behaviors (e.g., having sexual intercourse while not apparently awake, erratic driving, making incoherent phone calls).

The melatonin agonist, ramelteon (Rozerem®), does seem to improve sleep for some patients, and the drug is not associated with any known untoward effects. It is a good choice for the elderly, albeit with variable efficacy.

Stay away from older antidepressants (e.g., amitriptyline), diphenhydramine, haloperidol, and barbiturates in most patients (because of side effects) but especially in the elderly.

Restless Leg Syndrome (RLS)

Restless leg syndrome is a common sleep disorder in the elderly (prevalence = 20% in age > 80 years). The hallmark of RLS is leg discomfort +/– paresthesias at rest, relieved immediately with movement. Usually, pain is "deep seated" and localizes below the knees. Symptoms are worse in the evening and at night.

RLS can be primary or caused by other conditions: Iron deficiency (even without anemia), dialysis, diabetic neuropathy, multiple sclerosis, Parkinson's, pregnancy, and

others. Make sure that the patient's complaints aren't actually akathisias from medications (phenothiazines and SSRIs).

Diagnosis is made based on clinical history, a normal neuro exam, and absence of kidney disease. Always check a ferritin level to rule out iron deficiency, even if the patient does not have anemia.

The following expert panel recommendations are based on whether the RLS is intermittent, daily, or refractory.

- **Intermittent**: Try nonpharmacologic therapy first: Iron-replacement therapy; mental-alerting activities (such as video games or crosswords); avoidance of caffeine, nicotine, and alcohol.

  Then, if needed, try one of the following:
  ○ Dopamine agonists generally are the drugs of choice: pramipexole, ropinirole.
  ○ Levodopa. Be careful—may cause augmentation (worsen symptoms or rebound).
  ○ Benzodiazepines (generally avoided).
  ○ Low-potency opioids (generally avoided).
- **Daily**: Try nonpharmacologic first, then dopamine agonists, gabapentin, and, lastly, low-potency opioids.
- **Refractory** to dopamine agonists: Try gabapentin, a different dopamine agonist, combination therapy, then tramadol and, lastly, high-potency opioids.

Dizziness

Dizziness is common in the elderly but is not a normal consequence of aging. When any patient complains of "dizziness," take a good history (more sensitive in making the diagnosis than PE, labs, or studies) to determine which of the following she is actually describing:

- Vertigo: "Spinning," "whirling," or "moving" of either herself or the environment that is worse with head movement and occurs in spells (days to weeks), then eventually resolves.
- Nonspecific dizziness: Unable to characterize better; sometimes "lightheaded" is used to describe.
- Disequilibrium: Imbalance with standing and walking, especially with turning.
- Presyncope: Almost "fainting" or "blacking out" while either standing or seated (not supine), possibly associated with sweating, a sensation of warming, visual blurriness, and nausea.

A complete discussion about the workup of dizziness is included in the Neurology section. Multisensory deficits causing disequilibrium and benign positional vertigo are common. In geriatric patients, the cause is more often vestibular than in other patient groups.

The common causes of dizziness in the elderly usually can be discovered by history.

Presyncope. Dizziness that sounds like presyncope or "faintness" should be taken seriously and evaluated with a cardiovascular workup, especially if the patient has known heart disease, palpitations, or a history of true syncope.

Multisensory deficits. Think about multisensory deficits as a cause for disequilibrium in the patient with a mix of visual, hearing, orthopedic, and neuropathic impairments (sometimes also called "benign dysequilibrium of aging"). He complains of "feeling unsteady" and improves with a walker or when someone holds his arm. Treat this by maximizing support for each sensory impairment and providing assistance devices (e.g., canes, walkers).

Benign positional vertigo (BPV) presents as recurrent (lasts for weeks in spells), short-lived (< 1 minute), with episodes of vertigo that predominantly occur when the patient changes position. The vertigo can be bad enough to cause nausea and vomiting; but, otherwise, the patient has no other symptoms (e.g., hearing loss, headaches). Know that BPV occurs more often in geriatric patients who have giant cell arteritis (see the Rheumatology section), so take a good history in the dizzy elderly patient to determine whether symptoms of vasculitis or polymyalgia rheumatica are also present (e.g., weight loss, fevers, musculoskeletal pain).

In uncertain cases, BPV can be diagnosed by performing a maneuver in the office called the Dix-Hallpike test. This test turns the patient's head, then rapidly tilts her backwards for 30 seconds, then upright again, with subsequent observation for nystagmus. Repeat the maneuver with the head turned in the opposite direction. Visible nystagmus in either the recumbent or the upright position signals a positive test.

In these cases, the differential diagnosis includes central causes of vertigo such as cerebellar lesions (strokes or masses); so if the history is suggestive, do further workup with imaging and electronystagmography (water calorics).

Treatment of BPV can be accomplished through one of 2 office maneuvers, Epley and Semont, both equivalent in efficacy and designed to reposition the floating debris felt to be responsible for the vertigo. The maneuvers are variants of the Dix-Hallpike test, where you lean patients backwards and forwards with an associated neck tilt. Alternatively, exercises can be prescribed for home that aim to have the same result (but are less effective). No drugs are used to treat BPV.

CARDIOVASCULAR

Walking more than 4 hours per week is associated with a dramatic decrease in cardiovascular-related hospitalizations in persons > 65 years of age.

Isolated systolic hypertension is a common finding in elderly patients. It increases the risk of myocardial infarction and stroke 2–4x. Several studies show these patients benefit from treatment, so long as the diastolic pressure doesn't fall too low (< 60 mmHg).

In the elderly, start with about 1/2 the standard dose of any one of the following: Thiazides (chlorthalidone is now being favored over hydrochlorothiazide because of its superior efficacy and reduced rate of hypokalemia), dihydropyridine calcium-channel blockers (e.g., amlodipine), or ACE inhibitors/angiotensin II receptor blockers. Avoid beta-blockers for treatment of systolic hypertension in the elderly because they don't work as well as the other treatments and have been associated with increased mortality.

The 6-month mortality rate after an MI increases with age—from 4% around age 66 to 12% when older than 80 years (group = first MI, with thrombolytics, discharged from hospital). Only about 75% of eligible patients are receiving aspirin on discharge from the hospital. Be sure to prescribe an antiplatelet drug to these patients!

CHF. The incidence of congestive heart failure (CHF) in the elderly is increasing dramatically and is now the number 1 cause of hospitalizations in this group (number 2 is pneumonia).

Treat CHF itself primarily with diet, diuretics, and ACE inhibitors. Digoxin is indicated only for more severe heart failure. Isosorbide dinitrate and beta-blockers have an important secondary role. Use of NSAIDs is an important precipitant of CHF in older patients who already have risk factors for CHF.

Mortality benefit has been shown for ACE inhibitors, beta-blockers, and spironolactone. If you use spironolactone, follow K$^+$ closely. Spironolactone benefit has been shown in patients with class 4 CHF or class 3 with a history of class 4.

PULMONARY

Geriatric Asthma

Elderly patients with asthma may have long-standing asthma acquired in childhood/young adulthood, or they may have developed it as an aging adult. Around 8% of adults > age 65 are diagnosed with adult-onset asthma. Be aware that it is commonly misdiagnosed as COPD because COPD is more likely to occur in this age group.

Risks for development of adult-onset asthma are the same as for younger patients: allergens and irritants (tobacco smoke, occupational vapors, air pollution). Comorbidities are important, especially coronary heart disease, because treatment of asthma with beta-agonists can cause myocardial ischemia. Also, beta-blockers used as antihypertensive drugs can exacerbate airway obstruction.

Asthma in the older patient can present the same as in the younger patient, although elderly tend to have fewer symptoms with the same amount of disease. Specifically, they complain less of dyspnea associated with

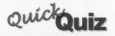

- What cause of dizziness is associated with improvement when the patient holds onto a walker?
- Which maneuver helps identify benign positional vertigo?
- What are the GOLD recommendations for diagnosis of asthma in the elderly?
- Is urinary incontinence considered a normal consequence of aging?
- What are the 4 types of incontinence?

obstruction and wheezing—likely due to their reduced activity, they fail to notice they are short of breath. Definitive diagnosis is made with spirometry, when the FEV_1 and FEV_1/FVC are reduced. In the elderly the traditional cut off of 70% for a diagnosis of obstruction, as recommended by the GOLD group (see the Pulmonary Medicine section on Asthma), is not used. This is due to the fact that this criterion is not as specific in this age group and will overdiagnose asthma! Instead, for diagnosis of asthma in the elderly, most experts use an $FEV_1/FVC < 89\%$ of the lower limit of normal for age. A response to bronchodilators is still expected, as per the GOLD criteria, for diagnosis: > 200 cc increase in FEV_1 post bronchodilator and > 12% of predicted.

Separating COPD from asthma is important, especially in the elderly where rates of COPD are high. Know that reversible obstruction is consistent with asthma, and a low DLCO is consistent with emphysematous COPD.

Bronchoprovocation is used to diagnose asthma in patients with normal spirometry, the same way as it is used in younger people.

Management of geriatric asthma is the same as for younger patients, but theophylline is not recommended, even as an alternative drug, because of the significant potential for toxicity.

Geriatric Sleep Apnea

Think about sleep apnea as a potential cause of reduced cognition in geriatric patients. Know that apnea which results in poor sleep and excessive daytime somnolence carries a higher rate of morbidity in patients who are frail and already prone to falls. Diagnosis and management is the same as in younger patients.

UROLOGY

Urinary Incontinence

Overview

Normal micturition is dependent on an intact neurologic pathway from the brainstem to the bladder, which causes relaxation of the sphincter muscle's tonic contractile state just milliseconds before contraction of the detrusor (bladder muscle). Additionally, voluntary control of micturition requires communication between the cerebral cortex and the brainstem.

Urinary incontinence, although a common geriatric problem, is always considered a pathologic condition that is not a normal consequence of aging! Always consider the possibility that the patient has a serious underlying condition responsible for the leakage.

Normal, age-related changes to the urinary tract include decreased flow rate, decreased bladder capacity, and increased residual volume. As a function of these changes, it is normal for patients to get up once during the night to void.

Urinary incontinence may be thought of as either a "storage problem" or an "outflow" problem. Storage problems are "detrusor" or bladder over- and under-contractility, while outflow problems are outlet obstruction or incompetence.

There are 4 general, symptom-based types of urinary incontinence:

1) **Urge** = Leakage (a lot or a little) associated with the feeling of urgency

2) **Stress** = Leakage associated with increased intraabdominal pressure (e.g., coughing, sneezing)

3) **Mixed** = Leakage associated with both an urgency and increased intraabdominal pressure

4) **Incomplete Bladder Emptying** = Leakage (a lot or a little) after voiding

Note that "overactive bladder" is not necessarily incontinence. It is a urologic condition defined by the urgent need to void frequently and during the middle of the night. Occasionally, the urgency may be associated with leakage, in which case, it is called urge incontinence (next).

Urge Incontinence

1) Urge incontinence (UI) is a common cause of geriatric incontinence. With urge incontinence, there is passage of either small or large amounts of urine, associated with a sense of urgency often set off by a precipitating stimulus: hearing running water, unlocking the door to the house, entering cold environments.

UI is related to overactive bladder.

UI and overactive bladders are caused by uncontrollable bladder contractions ("detrusor instability")—usually caused by CNS problems (termed "detrusor hyperreflexia"), but also sometimes a result of cystitis.

Detrusor hyperreflexia is due to progressive loss of communication between the frontal lobes and the micturition center in the brainstem. As the bladder loses the modulating influence from the brain, it tends to spasm more often.

Treatment is best accomplished with behavioral therapy, called bladder training. When an urge to void becomes profound, the patient is instructed to attempt relaxation techniques that help the urge subside and allows short-term voiding delay. Once the urge is controlled, the patient can walk calmly to the restroom and urinate. The goal is to eventually delay voiding to every 4 hours with no interval leakage.

Bladder training is more effective than the more commonly prescribed therapy of antimuscarinic agents (oxybutynin, tolterodine, fesoterodine, trospium, solifenacin, darifenacin, hyoscyamine, and tricyclic antidepressants), all of which are equivalent in efficacy and relax the bladder muscle. They have other anticholinergic side effects (e.g., dry mouth, tachycardia, constipation). Even so, these antimuscarinic agents are helpful when used as an adjunct to bladder training—short term, as needed. Remember that anticholinergics can precipitate acute angle glaucoma! Also do not use them for incontinence in patients who are taking cholinesterase inhibitors for dementia because the combination accelerates cognitive decline.

Pelvic muscle exercises (Kegel's) are also helpful for UI.

Stress Incontinence

2) Stress urinary incontinence (SUI) is second in frequency in geriatric women. With SUI, the urethra cannot maintain the pressure gradient required for urinary control when there is an increase in intraabdominal pressure (cough, jumping, etc.). SUI is associated with multiple vaginal deliveries, pelvic surgery, postmenopausal hormonal changes (low estrogen → atrophic relaxation of the vaginal wall → lack of support for the urethra) but is sometimes seen in males post-prostatectomy. Stress incontinence is initially best treated with behavioral therapy, especially Kegel exercises (perineal muscle contractions); referral to a pelvic floor physical therapy specialist can be helpful in effective teaching of Kegel's. Note that some women with urinary incontinence have a mixture of SUI and urge incontinence. Surgery has high cure rates but with high risk of complications. Periurethral collagen injections are an option for those who cannot have (or don't want) surgery and who do not improve with exercises.

The history gives you the clues to determine whether incontinence is due to urge or stress incontinence—look for the stimuli that precipitate leakage in a patient with UI and look for leakage associated with increased intraabdominal pressure with SUI.

Mixed Incontinence

3) Mixed incontinence, again, is a combination of urge and stress incontinence. The true etiology is unknown. Bladder training and Kegel's help these patients too.

Incomplete Emptying

4) Incomplete bladder emptying is sometimes still called "overflow incontinence." It is caused by either an overactive bladder +/– an outlet obstruction or by an underactive bladder that has trouble contracting (e.g., diabetes, Parkinson's, alcohol abuse).

Although rare in females, incomplete emptying in males is usually caused by prostatic hypertrophy. The outlet obstruction causes a distended bladder and high-volume, post-void retention. Anticholinergic drugs are the most common causes of drug-induced incomplete emptying. Psychogenic retention can also be a cause.

Most types of incomplete emptying do indeed cause urgency and may be seen as a type of urge incontinence.

Treatment includes alpha-blockers for men with benign prostatic hypertrophy (BPH).

Review

• Bladder training and Kegel exercises: Urge, stress, and mixed
• Drugs for urge and mixed (anticholinergics with antimuscarinic effects): Oxybutynin, tolterodine, trospium, solifenacin, darifenacin
• Drugs for stress: None! Bladder training and Kegel's only!
• Surgery: Last resort for stress
• Incomplete emptying: Treat underlying cause if possible; intermittent catheterization; "diaper-like" garments

Know that asymptomatic bacteriuria, while common in the elderly, is not a cause of incontinence. Also know that incontinence is never an indication for a long-term bladder catheter.

Fecal Incontinence

Geriatric fecal incontinence is usually caused by fecal impaction and secondary overflow incontinence. The impaction is usually a result of lax muscles and neuronal degeneration. Typical presentation is an elderly person with complaints of diarrhea and abdominal discomfort and who has hard stool in the rectal vault on physical exam. Treatment is disimpaction and subsequent bulking agents.

Benign Prostatic Hyperplasia (BPH)

The prevalence of benign prostatic hyperplasia (BPH) increases from about 10% at age 30 to > 80% at age 85; about 15% of these patients have impaired urination. We still don't understand what causes BPH and have yet to identify any specific risk factors—except age. BPH does not increase the chance of prostate cancer.

Symptoms of BPH are fairly specific for urinary retention: frequency, hesitancy, difficulty starting and stopping the stream, urgency, and nocturia. Certainly other

Quick Quiz

- What is the best treatment for urge incontinence?
- What is the best initial treatment for stress urinary incontinence?
- What is a common cause for incomplete bladder emptying in males?
- What is the role of bladder catheterization in the treatment of geriatric incontinence?
- How does prostatic hyperplasia affect PSA levels?
- What is the initial treatment for BPH?
- What is the most common cause of neurogenic ED?

diseases can cause these symptoms (e.g., bladder cancer, cystitis) and should be considered before making a diagnosis of BPH.

The 2 definitive tests that should be done: a digital rectal exam to palpate the prostate and assess for irregularities and increased size; and, a urinalysis to assess for hematuria (with a culture if infection is suspected). Know that serum prostate-specific antigen (PSA) levels increase as the prostate increases in size, so PSA screening for prostate cancer is less specific in men with BPH (more false positives).

BPH is treated only if it significantly affects the patient adversely and/or if it is associated with outlet obstruction, causing hydronephrosis or acute kidney injury.

Treatment starts with medical therapy: alpha-blockers (terazosin, doxazosin, tamsulosin, alfuzosin, silodosin) or 5-alpha-reductase inhibitors (finasteride, dutasteride).

Note: Of the alpha-blockers, prazosin is not used for BPH because it requires frequent doses and has more side effects.

Most common side effects of these meds are orthostasis and dizziness. Be careful with combining sildenafil or vardenafil with these drugs because the combination worsens hypotension.

The 5-alpha-reductase inhibitors, which reduce circulating testosterone, take at least 6 months to decrease prostate size and relieve symptoms. These drugs work better for large prostates and have a more durable effect. The major side effect is impairment of sexual function (decreased libido and delayed ejaculation). Know that these drugs decrease serum PSA, even in cancer patients, so recommendations are to multiply the measured PSA by 2–2.5, depending on how long the patient has been taking the drug.

Transurethral resection of the prostate (TURP) is now the treatment of last resort, used when drugs fail to work.

Other guidance: Make sure patients know to reduce intake of caffeine and alcohol (diuretics), stay away from fluids before bed, and attempt to urinate twice to completely empty the bladder.

Erectile Dysfunction (Impotence)

Overview

The most common type of male sexual dysfunction is erectile dysfunction (ED), which is defined as the inability to achieve or maintain an erection sufficient for satisfactory sexual intercourse. It is not uncommon for men to experience brief episodes of ED. "Impotence" is the term reserved for ED that occurs in > 75% of sexual encounters.

The smooth muscle in the flaccid penis is in a state of tonus or contraction due to alpha stimulation by norepinephrine. cGMP is made, along with cAMP—made by the norepinephrine and vasoactive intestinal peptide (VIP) pathways. This cGMP causes the relaxation of the smooth muscle in the penis, which increases the inflow through the helicine artery into the erectile tissue. The swelling of this tissue causes compression of the outflow venules, resulting in a sustained erection.

ED can be caused by organic or psychological problems, or as a side effect of medications (25% of cases!). Most causes of ED are at least partially organic. The organic causes are neurogenic, vascular, hormonal, and normal aging.

Classic Presentations and Causes of ED

There are many causes of ED. These can be grouped as follows:

- **Organic causes**: Usually slow onset. Loss of nocturnal and morning erections.

  - **Neurogenic**: Usual cause is diabetes. Other causes are surgical procedures (especially prostate), MS, ALS, Parkinson's, and other causes of peripheral neuropathy. Cyclists who spend > 3 hours/week on an upright bicycle can experience ED due to pressure that the seat places on the pudendal nerves (reducing blood flow to cavernosal artery).

  - **Vascular**: Usual cause is diabetes and/or cardiovascular disease. Other causes are surgical procedures, inflammatory conditions, or pelvic fracture. In elderly men, ED is caused by vascular compromise in 50% (indicated by a low penile brachial pressure index [PBPI]). ED due to vascular compromise indicates increased risk of present and future major vascular disease.

  - **Hormonal**: Often accompanied by a loss of libido. Symptoms may include gradual onset of frontal headaches or visual disturbances (space-occupying tumor); hot flashes and decreased need for shaving (decreased androgens); fatigue + weight gain + dry skin + constipation (hypothyroidism).

∘ **Normal aging**: Sexual potency does decrease with age.

• **Medications**: Especially antidepressants (SSRIs), clonidine, spironolactone, beta-blockers, and thiazide diuretics. Many others also cause ED, but these are some of the most commonly prescribed meds in the geriatric population.

• **Psychogenic**: Usually acute onset. This is the usual cause for ED in younger patients. They continue to have nocturnal and morning erections, but libido is lost. ED is directly correlated with depression. Unfortunately, SSRIs are associated with a very high incidence of sexual dysfunction (usually delayed ejaculation).

Treatment Options for ED

First-Line Treatment for ED [Know]:

Sildenafil citrate (Viagra®) inhibits phosphodiesterase type 5 (PDE5), an enzyme that inactivates cGMP. It works very well for many causes of ED. Side effects are due to its vasodilatory properties—headaches, flushing, dyspepsia, bluish hue in the vision. Contraindications are any concurrent nitrates. Relative contraindications are CHF, hypotension, unstable angina, HCM, and severe aortic stenosis.

Vardenafil (Levitra®) is similar in mechanism, effectiveness, and side effects to sildenafil.

Tadalafil (Cialis®) has the same mechanism of action as sildenafil and vardenafil but with a longer half-life. Erectile function may be improved for up to 36 hours. This drug is approved for daily use. One specific side effect is back pain.

PDE5 inhibitors are more likely to cause hypotension when taken with non-selective alpha blockers (prazosin, doxazosin, and terazosin). Uroselective alpha blockers (tamsulosin and alfuzosin) are less likely to cause hypotension. There is a risk of hearing loss with all of the PDE5 inhibitors.

Vacuum devices work well but are clumsy to use. They are indicated only when oral therapy is contraindicated or the patient prefers them to oral therapy.

Yohimbine is a naturally occurring alpha-blocker. It has minimal effect but, because it is inexpensive and has minimal side effects, it is often tried on patients with a mostly psychogenic etiology. Better than placebo but much less effective than sildenafil.

Second-Line Treatment for ED:

Alprostadil (prostaglandin E1) injected into the corpora cavernosa of the penis works well. It is especially useful in patients with ED due to neurologic dysfunction.

Third-Line Treatment:

Penile implants. Various types—hydraulic, semirigid, and flexible rods. Usually used only for those who have failed all other therapy. Complications are associated with the surgery. There is a risk of postsurgical infection. Scarring may cause erections to curve. Tissue erosion may occur. If there are no complications, they are effective and patient satisfaction rates are high.

HEARING

Decreased hearing is age-related. About 1/3 of patients > 65 years of age have hearing loss. The most common cause is presbycusis, which is just age-related sensorineural hearing loss. It is bilateral, and loss of higher frequency sounds is more common. Be sure to check for cerumen impaction. See other causes of decreased hearing on page 10-44. Hearing aids can help these patients.

ETHICS

OVERVIEW

Read the ACP's Ethics Manual, 5th edition (released 2005), available online at www.acponline.org/ethics/ethicman.htm

PHYSICIAN'S DUTY AND PATIENT'S RIGHTS

The physician's duty to the patient is based on 3 principles that are the basis for all ethical physician-patient interaction:

1) Beneficence—the duty to act in the best interests and welfare of the patient and the health of society
2) Nonmaleficence—the duty to do no harm to the patient
3) Respect for the patient's autonomy—helping the patient make free, non-coerced choices

Let's look at specifics.

The patient's right to accept or refuse health care is based on another 3 principles:

1) The philosophical concept of personal autonomy—a value held close to the heart in our culture
2) Personal liberty interest under the Constitution
3) Common law right of self-determination

Patients should be able to choose and follow their own ideas and plans for their life. Constraint of a person's free choices is permissible only when these choices infringe on another person's rights and welfare. Paternalism, the practice of overriding or ignoring preferences of patients in order to benefit them, used to be the standard of interaction between the physician and patient. Today, except for certain cases (mental illness and some emergencies), paternalism is considered ethically improper. Patients should be an active part of the decision-making process. Patients require informed consent, which is defined as the willing acceptance of medical intervention—after

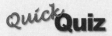

Quick Quiz

- Which medications most commonly cause erectile dysfunction?

- If an exam presents a young male with erectile dysfunction who is on no medications, what is the most likely etiology?

- What is the mechanism of action for sildenafil?

- Name a scenario in which a physician can ethically have a sexual relationship with a patient.

- What is the difference between an advanced directive and a living will?

adequate disclosure by the physician—of the nature of the intervention and all of its risks and benefits.

Patients are entitled to disclosure of the following:

1) The patient's current medical status with the probable course, whether or not medical intervention is used
2) The medical interventions that may help and the risks associated with them
3) The physician's opinion about other alternatives
4) The physician's own recommendations based on best clinical judgment

Know that physicians are responsible for caring for patients with contagious infectious diseases. It is deemed unethical by ACP for internists to refuse care for patients with HIV/AIDS, hepatitis viruses, multidrug resistant TB, and influenza because of a physician's own fear of becoming infected. It is assumed that the physician will take appropriate infection control precautions.

Know that physicians are responsible for providing honest information on disability claim forms and should not attempt to erroneously assist a patient in obtaining disability.

Generally, physicians should avoid caring for close family members and friends.

It is absolutely unethical for physicians to have any sexual relationship with a current patient, regardless of who initiates the relationship. The ethics document from the Federation of State Medical Boards says that physicians cannot even have sexual relationships with the relatives of existing patients.

Even former patients can cause ethical problems. The ACP ethics document says that physicians should "consult with a colleague or other professional before becoming sexually involved with a former patient."

DISCONTINUING PATIENT RELATIONSHIPS

Physicians can sever relationships with patients so long as care is available by another physician (anywhere else), and the patient's health is not sacrificed. The physician must give the patient written notice of intent and must request approval from the patient for transfer of her medical records to the accepting physician. If this process is not followed, legal action can be taken for physician "abandonment."

MEDICAL RECORDS

The physical chart belongs to the hospital or physician, but the information in the chart belongs to the patient. If requested, you must release the entire chart to the patient, and you cannot hold the chart hostage in exchange for payment of services. However, it is legal to charge a reasonable fee for copies.

ADVANCED DIRECTIVE

The advanced directive is the means patients have for stating which treatments they would accept or decline if they lost decision-making capacity. The advanced directive may also specify general goals for medical care and the patient's choice of a surrogate—a person with durable power of attorney for the patient's health care.

A living will is a more focused form of advanced directive, in which the patient, for example, refuses life support when in a terminal condition. A lawyer is not needed to make a living will.

The patient has a right to change his/her mind! "Joe" has a living will. If he comes into the Emergency Department and requires intubation to survive—and states that he has changed his mind and wants all possible treatments available—then you honor his current decision.

Know that fluids and nutrition are ethically regarded as the same as other forms of treatment, and patients can address the desire for discontinuation of nutrition and fluids in their advanced directives.

PATIENT'S COMPETENCY OR DECISION-MAKING CAPACITY

The decision-making capacity refers to the ability to comprehend, evaluate, and choose among realistic options. The decision-making capacity of the patient can be difficult to determine. There are many transitory or reversible conditions that can interfere with this capacity. Examples are anxiety, depression, drug-induced confusion, and abnormal metabolic states. The waxing and waning associated with certain conditions, such as organic brain syndrome, is a manifestation of pathology, and the patient should be considered to have impaired capacity.

SURROGATE

A "surrogate" or "proxy" is a person who is authorized to make decisions on behalf of an incapacitated person. Traditionally, the next of kin has been considered the natural surrogate. In some states, there is a well-defined list of the order of next of kin, with priority given to natural surrogates—e.g., spouse, then parents, then children, then siblings. Another option is for the subject to give someone durable power of attorney. This means giving decision-making authorization to a person who supersedes family members. Remember: The "contract for health care" is between the physician and the patient, not the patient's family.

The surrogate's decisions must promote the patient's wishes and welfare. If the patient has expressed certain wishes on a topic regarding medical intervention in the past, the surrogate must use that knowledge in the decision-making process. If the surrogate has no knowledge of the patient's wishes, then the surrogate must make decisions based on the patient's welfare. Welfare should include consideration of suffering, preservation of life, restoration of function, and quality of life; decisions should be based on what a reasonable person would want in similar circumstances. The surrogates' authority ends when the patient dies (e.g., they are not able to give consent for autopsy).

EMERGENCY SITUATIONS

For patients unable to express their preferences, the physician may perform life-sustaining emergency procedures under the presumption that the alternative would be death or severe disability. All states have statutes allowing the physician to hold patients with certain psychiatric conditions against their will for medical and/or psychiatric treatment. This is often called a "medical hold."

QUALITY OF LIFE AND PAIN RELIEF IN PALLIATIVE CARE

The quality of life in terminally ill patients in pain is considerably improved by proper pain relief. Terminal patients in pain are in a special situation, and their requests for pain meds generally should be honored. The downside of pain medications is that they can cause confusion and a decreased ability to communicate. You have to strike a balance between maximum pain relief and minimal decrease in consciousness. The assistance of hospice workers in this situation can be very helpful.

PHYSICIAN ERROR

Physicians must disclose to the patient any errors in judgment and procedure when the information is deemed "material to the patient's well-being." In general, you always disclose errors—disclosure is not equivalent to admitting neglect.

PHYSICIAN-ASSISTED SUICIDE

The latest guidelines by the ACP and the AMA prohibit any form of physician assistance with suicide.

CPR AND DNR

Cardiopulmonary resuscitation (CPR) is usually a standing order in a hospital; i.e., it is to be carried out, without specific order, on any patient who suffers cardiac or respiratory arrest. The only time CPR is not done is when there is an order stating such—a "do not resuscitate" (DNR) or "do not attempt resuscitation" (DNAR) or "No Code" order. The decision about non-resuscitation has 3 considerations that must be assessed:

1) Whether or not CPR would be futile; i.e., that the resuscitation would be unlikely to succeed or, if it did, another cardiac or respiratory arrest would soon follow.
2) The preferences of the patient.
3) Expected quality of life of the patient if resuscitation succeeds. It is the responsibility of the physician to initiate discussions with the patient (or, if the patient is incompetent, with family members or a surrogate) who is terminally ill or has an incurable disease with an estimated 50% survival of less than 3 years. The attending physician should clearly write the "do not resuscitate" order on the order sheet in the patient's chart. The progress notes should detail the facts and opinions leading to that decision.

SUICIDE ATTEMPTS

Suicide attempts should always be treated despite the wishes of the patient. These patients are often "crying for help." They are also often in a pathological mental state that may be transitory or treatable. This situation is different from the patient who refuses life-sustaining treatment. The difference is that with refusal of care, the patients are not killing themselves—rather, they're refusing help that would keep them alive (uh, okay).

CULTURAL DIFFERENCES

A patient from another country/culture can present some ethical dilemmas. If family members of your elderly patient state a wish that their grandmother not be told about a terminal illness such as cancer, you can explain to your patient that she is very sick and ask whether she wishes to make these decisions or prefers to have them made by another. If the wish is the result of a particular custom, the patient often will want others to make the decisions. This can then be considered an authorized delegation of decision-making authority. If the patient says she wants to know everything and make her own decisions, you must side with the patient.

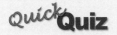

Quick Quiz

- 6 months ago, Mr. Jones, a man with terminal cancer, decided to invoke a living will that said he refuses all life support in case of cardiopulmonary arrest. Today, he presents to the ED in severe distress and says he wants everything done, including intubation. His family doesn't want anything done, and you have the signed living will at the bedside. What should you do now that his personal preference has changed in the face of a signed living will and family wishes for nothing to be done?

- You see a colleague drinking shots in a bar shortly before his 12-hour shift in the ED. Are you obligated to inform anyone?

CONFIDENTIALITY AND PUBLIC WELFARE

The personal and medical information that a physician obtains from a patient is (ethically and legally) confidential. But! In general, if the condition or disease of a patient can endanger other persons, the physician is legally and ethically obligated to report the situation to the appropriate parties. Many specifics are straightforward and are addressed with legal statutes. Common examples are sexually transmitted diseases and conditions that could affect the operator of a motor vehicle, such as seizures and severe cardiac arrhythmias. Others are more difficult. A patient with a serious, highly infectious disease (TB, meningococcemia) should not be allowed to infect others. These patients can be held against their will if their behavior is considered a threat to others. Some infectious diseases may necessitate informing the patient's employer (health-care worker, food worker, etc.).

Adolescents are allowed to consent for some services without parental involvement in some states. Know the laws of your own state in this regard. Adolescent consent for contraception is protected under federal law by language in the federal budget that restricts individual states from passing teen contraceptive laws, if that state receives federal subsidies for health care. So adolescent consent for birth control is acceptable in all states. Consent for abortion services, however, is state-dependent.

BRAIN DEATH

Physicians may stop treatment if a person is "brain dead" (loss of entire brain function, including brain stem). An EEG is not required for diagnosis. Organs can then be donated without patient's prior consent if the next of kin (or surrogate) gives permission, knowing that the patient would want that.

PHYSICIAN-PHYSICIAN vs. PUBLIC WELFARE OBLIGATIONS

The physician should not allow any incompetent or unethical conduct by other physicians. If you know of such conduct, the evidence should be presented to the appropriate authority. This may be the division chief or ethics committee of the hospital. Most state and many county medical societies now have confidential treatment of impaired physicians. Physicians who strongly suspect another physician is chemically impaired are obligated to urge the physician to seek treatment. If this impairment may affect medical competence, the obligation is to report the "credible evidence" to the local medical society. Note that a physician cannot act only on hearsay, but must have credible evidence before reporting it.

DRUG RESEARCH

It is unethical to use socioeconomic differences in choosing patients for a drug study, unless the socioeconomic status is considered a variable. For example, you cannot ethically test a drug only on those who can pay for it. Conversely, you cannot ethically offer a free drug for research only to those in a lower socioeconomic status.

FINANCIAL CONFLICTS

The ACP ethics document is very clear that certain financial relationships are unethical:

- The physician must disclose to patients if he intends to refer them to a facility or research study in which the physician has a financial stake.
- The physician should not refer patients to a care facility where she holds a financial interest but is not employed.
- A physician may not pay another physician for referrals.
- A physician may not receive payment or gifts (even "small ones") from device manufacturers or pharmaceutical companies for recommending or using their products.
- Physicians should not sell products out of their offices, unless they are meeting an unmet need of the community (e.g., selling crutches or walkers in a small town). Physicians should not sell supplements or cosmetics out of their offices.
- Physicians should not advertise using unsubstantiated or false statements nor should they omit necessary information.
- Physicians can and should act as expert witnesses to benefit society, but they cannot accept payment in exchange for biased testimony. Fees charged should be for "reasonable time and expenses."

SCENARIOS

Some scenarios:

1) A patient enters the hospital unconscious and near death with a terminal disease. What should the physician do if:

   a) The patient has a properly executed living will that states no intubation, CPR, etc.

   b) The patient has no living will, but family members say they strongly prefer the patient be allowed to die with dignity and without heroics.

   c) Same as "a)" but family members (many of whom are lawyers) say they want all possible heroic measures to be done—and threaten dire consequences if their wishes are not followed!

2) A patient comes to the ED with an extensive acute MI, is mentally competent, and refuses to be admitted despite being fully informed of the possible consequences. What do you do?

3) A respirator-dependent patient requests in writing to be extubated. What do you do?

4) A female health-care worker who is found to have hepatitis B antigen positivity requests that you not tell her supervisor at the hospital where she works.

5) A man is diagnosed with inoperable metastatic cancer. He states to his physician that he does not want his wife to know.

6) A newly married man just finds out that he has a serious autosomal dominant genetic disease such as Huntington disease. He requests that the physician not tell his wife.

7) A man finds out he is HIV-positive and requests that you not tell his spouse.

8) A woman with suspected meningococcal meningitis refuses to be admitted and wants to go back to work.

Answers:

1) The physician should:

   a) Follow instructions in the living will.

   b) In this situation the physician needs more information; needs to know the wishes of the patient, not the family!

   c) Follow instructions in the living will; the contract is between you and the patient. Besides, so far, all living wills have upheld in court.

2) You must show caring for the patient's situation, yet attempt to dissuade the patient from leaving. If the patient still leaves, it is prudent to have the patient sign out "AMA"—against medical advice (the patient is not legally required to do this). You cannot stop patients from leaving unless you think they are mentally incompetent or a danger to others (e.g., they want to drive home).

3) You need more information (mentally competent, fully informed, etc.). This is a problem with probable far-reaching consequences—not just for you, but for the patient's other doctors, the hospital, and the patient's family. First step is to contact the hospital's ethics committee. You may also need assistance from the patient's other doctors, family, psychiatry, and social services.

4) This health-care worker has a direct obligation not to cause harm to the patients with whom she interacts. If she refuses to inform the hospital infection control team, then you are obligated to do so.

5) Although the physician can strongly encourage the man of his wife's moral right to know the situation, communicating this to the spouse is ultimately the patient's obligation and not the physician's.

6) In this case, the physician should first strongly encourage the man to tell his wife. If that fails, the last resort is for the physician to tell the wife because of the risk of harm to future children.

7) In all HIV cases, the physician must make sure that anybody at risk (e.g., through sexual contact or IV drugs) is notified. Whenever patients say they are going to do the notification, the physician must ensure it is done. Usually, this obligation is taken care of by the state health department.

8) This patient may be held against her will for the good of public welfare.

PREOPERATIVE CARDIAC EVALUATION

Preoperative evaluation of a patient to determine the risks of having a cardiac event in the perioperative period is a topic you must know. There have been several guidelines produced by different medical societies. As of this writing, the AHA/ACC "Guidelines for Perioperative Cardiovascular Evaluation for Noncardiac Surgery" is the most recent document, with a focused update in 2009 regarding the use of perioperative beta-blockers to minimize intraoperative cardiac risk.

These guidelines recommend 5 steps to be followed:

Step 1: Does the patient need emergency noncardiac surgery? If so, then the patient should proceed to surgery; perioperative surveillance and postoperative risk stratification and risk-factor management should proceed as best as possible.

If the answer is no, this is not emergent and proceed to Step 2.

Step 2: Does the patient have an active cardiac condition?

• Unstable coronary syndrome (unstable or severe angina or recent MI, defined as more than 7 days but ≤ 1 month)

• Decompensated heart failure

• Significant arrhythmias: 3rd degree AV block, Mobitz II AV block, symptomatic ventricular arrhythmias, supraventricular arrhythmias (includes atrial fib!)

- Know all of the scenarios in the ethics topic!
- What type of preoperative evaluation is done if a patient requires emergent noncardiac surgery?
- Know the 5-step process used in determining if a patient requires a pre-op cardiac evaluation.

with uncontrolled ventricular rate (> 100 bpm at rest), symptomatic bradycardia, new ventricular tachycardia
- Severe valvular disease: Any symptomatic aortic stenosis, asymptomatic aortic stenosis with gradient greater than 40 mmHg, symptomatic mitral stenosis

If so, then the patient should undergo evaluation and treatment before noncardiac surgery.

If these are not present, proceed to Step 3.

Step 3: Is the patient undergoing low-risk surgery? Here, the guideline gets murky. It is definite with defining very low-risk as superficial and ophthalmologic procedures, and the highest-risk as major vascular procedures. It lists endovascular abdominal aortic aneurysm repair and carotid endarterectomy as intermediate-risk. After listing these specifically, it goes on to state: "The physician must exercise judgment to correctly access perioperative surgical risks and the need for further evaluation." Wow, thanks guideline … In general, though, any procedure that is "ambulatory" in nature and does not require "hospital admission" is usually considered low-risk. Other surgeries in this category include all breast surgeries and endoscopic procedures.

So, if you get to Step 3 and the surgery is low risk, proceed with surgery; if not, go to Step 4.

Step 4: Does the patient have good functional capacity without symptoms? If this is true, proceed with moderate- to high-risk surgery.

What is a simple, easy method to assess functional capacity? The guideline recommends using a MET level of ≥ 4. Now let's review that "MET" thing again. Remember that functional capacity can be expressed as metabolic equivalents (METs); 1 MET is the resting or basal oxygen consumption of a 70-kg, 40-year-old man in a resting state. Functional capacity is classified as excellent (> 10 METs), good (7–10 METs), moderate (4–7 METs), poor (< 4 METs), or unknown. Think of 4 METs as equivalent to carrying groceries up the stairs. Examples associated with < 4 METs include slow ballroom dancing, golfing with a cart, and walking at a speed of 2–3 mph. Activities that require > 4 METs include moderate cycling, climbing hills, skiing, singles tennis, and jogging. There are several scales (e.g., Duke Activity Status, Specific Activity Scale) out there, but, in general, this guide will help you.

So if the patient can run up a hill or mow his lawn without problems, then he likely can proceed with his planned surgery. If he can't, then we go to Step 5.

Step 5: Here, we have the patient who has gotten to step 5 because of either poor or unknown functional capacity, and we must use clinical risk factors to help us determine if he can proceed to surgery.

The 5 clinical risk factors to ask about:

1) History of ischemic heart disease (history of MI + exercise stress test, current chest pain, nitrate use, ECG with pathologic Qs)
2) Heart failure history (prior or compensated)
3) Cerebrovascular disease history
4) Diabetes
5) Renal insufficiency (creatinine > 2 mg/dL)

If the patient has 1 or 2 risk factors, proceed with planned surgery with heart rate controlled with beta-blockers (best if started almost 30 days before surgery and with a pulse rate of 55–60 as goal) or consider testing if it will change management.

If > 3 risk factors are present, the surgery-specific risk is important (Table 10-9 on next page). The guidelines say, for "… intermediate-risk surgery, there are insufficient data to determine the best strategy (proceeding with planned surgery with tight heart rate control with beta blockade or further cardiovascular testing if it will change management)."

Bottom line: Aortic, major vascular surgery or peripheral vascular surgery generally requires further cardiac evaluation. Low-risk procedures (endoscopic, superficial, cataracts, breast surgery, or any ambulatory surgery) do not. Intermediate … it's up to your judgment.

Scenarios you are likely to encounter:

- A low-risk patient who can proceed directly to surgery of any type without noninvasive testing
- A moderate-risk patient with good functional capacity who can go directly to a non-vascular surgery
- A major-risk patient who needs further workup as defined in the charts prior to going to surgery

Beta-blockers: Know that high-dose beta-blockers used perioperatively, given without a history of dose titration, in beta-blocker-naive patients do reduce primary cardiac events but carry an increased risk of mortality and stroke—hence, they are not recommended.

Who gets beta-blockers?

- Vascular surgery patients with positive pre-op stress tests.
- Continue these in patients already receiving them for angina, arrhythmias, or HTN.

Table 10-9: Risk of Procedure; AHA/ACC	
Low Risk	Endoscopies, local biopsies, breast biopsies, vasectomy, cataract surgery
Intermediate Risk	Surgeries: Carotid endarterectomy, intraperitoneal, intrathoracic, orthopedic, prostate, head and neck
Major Risk	Surgeries: Aortic and major vascular, cardiothoracic, emergent major surgery, long procedures with large blood loss and/or fluid shifts

PRE-OP SCREENING LABS

General guidelines follow, and are based on, an amalgam of various societies' recommendations!

Hematocrit:

• > 65 years of age for major surgery
• All surgeries that will/could result in major blood loss
• Not for minor surgery!
• CBC is not recommended unless cheaper than hematocrit alone

Electrolytes: Not recommended unless history suggests reason to check.

Creatinine:

• > 50 years of age
• Major surgery
• Hypotension is likely
• Nephrotoxic drugs to be used

Glucose, liver function tests, PT/PTT, U/A: Not recommended unless clinical signs/symptoms warrant.

ECG:

• Yes for all vascular procedures
• Nonvascular procedures:
  ◦ Men > 45 years
  ◦ Women > 55 years
  ◦ Known cardiac disease
  ◦ Clinical evaluation suggests possible cardiac disease
  ◦ Diuretic use (electrolyte abnormality possible)
  ◦ DM, hypertension, renal insufficiency
  ◦ Major surgical procedure

CXR:

• > 50 years of age for major surgery
• Suspected cardiac or pulmonary disease

PFTs:

• Not recommended for healthy patients prior to any surgery
• Use for dyspnea that is unexplained

Stents and such: Hold off on elective noncardiac surgery if:

• Within 4–6 weeks of bare-metal stent placement
• Within 12 months of drug-eluting stent if patient must stop thienopyridine/aspirin
• Within 4 weeks of balloon angioplasty

PREVENTIVE MEDICINE

PATIENT EDUCATION

[Know this entire topic. Consider all of Patient Education highlighted]

Because patient education improves outcomes, periodically review and counsel patients on the following:

• Tobacco
• Firearms
• Alcohol/substance abuse
• Physical activity level
• Obesity

Check the elderly for functional status, gait abnormalities, and for osteoporosis risk factors.

Teach males about self-examination of the testes.

Guide all patients about self-examination for skin disease, gum disease, STDs, and nutrition.

Recommend seat belts and good fluid intake.

Got all that?

Teaching women to perform a breast self-exam does not reduce their mortality from breast cancer, so most organizations are no longer recommending it.

Firearm-related injury and death is a major public health problem. The physician's ethical role is to counsel patients about firearm safety and become involved in community efforts to prevent firearm injuries.

Smoking cessation

Tobacco smoke is responsible for 90% of all lung cancer deaths and more than 10% of cardiovascular deaths.

The Agency for Health Care Policy and Research (AHCPR) Smoking Cessation Clinical Practice Guideline (2008 Update): At each patient visit, ask about tobacco products. The AHCPR guideline even recommends that tobacco usage be added as the fifth "vital sign." If the patient smokes, give strong, clear, personalized antismoking counseling. If the patient is willing to quit, set a "quit date" (preferably within 2 weeks), recommend pharmacologic therapy (see below), provide personal or group counseling, and schedule a follow-up visit. Tell discouraged smokers that most previous smokers required many (> 5) attempts to quit.

Know that cessation of smoking can exacerbate ulcerative colitis.

First-line medications for anti-smoking:

• Bupropion SR
• Nicotine (gum, inhaler, lozenges, nasal spray, patch)
• Varenicline (Chantix®)

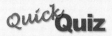

- Which patients are started on beta-blockers before surgery?
- Know the pre-op screening labs and who gets them.
- What patient education topics should you review and counsel patients about periodically?

Counseling + meds: Better than counseling alone.

Varenicline is a partial agonist of nicotinic acetylcholine receptors and is associated with serious neuropsychiatric side effects (behavior changes, suicidal ideation and behavior, and depressed mood).

Note that cigar smoking increases the risk of coronary heart disease (relative risk = 1.27), COPD (1.45), and cancers of the mouth and throat (2.02).

Other Disease Risks

Increases risk of disease:

- High intake of red meat increases risk of colorectal cancer.
- Alcohol increases risk of colon, breast, esophageal, and oropharyngeal cancers.
- Obesity is associated with increased risk of colon, breast, endometrial, kidney, and esophageal cancers—and may increase risk for prostate, ovary and cervix, liver and gall bladder, and pancreatic cancers, myeloma, and lymphoma! (Is there anything left?)
- Bladder cancer is inversely associated with fluid intake. Incidence in the high fluid-intake group is half that of those in the low fluid-intake group.
- Organisms that cause or increase the risk of cancer: HPV, HBV, HCV, HIV, EBV, and *H. pylori*.

Decreases risk of disease:

- High intake of tomatoes decreases prostate cancer risk.
- Fiber reduces heart disease and diabetes. Not sure about cancer, though.
- Vitamin D may decrease colorectal and prostate cancer risk.

Note that supplemental vitamins and minerals do not decrease cancer risk in patients with adequate diets.

Certain drugs are used to decrease cancer risks in special patient populations:

- Tamoxifen and raloxifene decrease breast cancer.
- NSAIDs and aspirin decrease colon polyps and colon cancer.

- Dutasteride (and probably finasteride) decreases prostate cancer.

SCREENING EXAMS

Overview

Screening protocols: Table 10-10 provides a rough summary.

Every official entity detailing screening protocols has a different, but usually similar, suggested protocol for each disease. In the following, abbreviations used are:

ACP = American College of Physicians

ACS = American Cancer Society

NCI = National Cancer Institute

USPSTF = U.S. Preventive Services Task Force

Cardiovascular Disease

Blood Pressure and Cholesterol

Blood pressure: Every 2 years and every clinical encounter.

Cholesterol: Screen men 35–65 years old and women 45–65 years old every 5 years. If the patient is placed on lipid-lowering agents, then generally they are checked every 6 months to a year thereafter. If the screening total cholesterol is near the threshold, it should be repeated periodically. See the Endocrinology section for treatment.

The Endocrinology section also discusses the recommendations for lipid screening contained in the latest document from the National Cholesterol Education Panel (NCEP), entitled Adult Treatment Panel III (with the relevant Update from 2004). NCEP is an advisory group

Table 10-10: Screening Exam Recommendations

Counseling about smoking	Each visit
Counseling, other	Initial visit and then periodically*
Blood Pressure	Each visit; at least every 2 years
Cholesterol	Every 5 years is appropriate
Breast Exams	Controversial*
Mammograms	Yearly after age 50*
Digital Rectal Exam	Yearly after age 50
FOBT	Yearly after age 50 (not needed after colonoscopy)
Colonoscopy	See GI section, page 1-32
Pap Smear	Every 3 years*
PSA	Inconclusive*
* See text for more information	

formed out of the National Heart Lung and Blood Institute (NHLBI), which is a subset of NIH (as is NCI). The ATP III (and Update) screening recommendations vary slightly from the ones listed above but not by much.

The same situation is true for BP recommendations contained in the latest document from the Joint National Committee on Prevention, Detection, Evaluation, and Treatment of High Blood Pressure (JNC 7, 2003)—also an NHLBI advisory group. We discuss JNC7 in the Nephrology section. Again, slight differences.

Both ATP III and JNC 7 are due for an updated release in 2011.

Estimating Cardiovascular Risk

For patients who do not currently have heart disease but have at least 2 risk factors for heart disease (per NCEP ATP III criteria—see the Endocrinology section), know to estimate their 5-year, 10-year, or lifetime risk for heart disease using one of the many established risk predictor models (e.g., Framingham Risk Assessment). The result gives you good insight into how aggressive you need to be about reducing their cardiovascular risk factors.

Diabetes

The American Diabetes Association (ADA) recommends annual screening with a venous fasting plasma glucose (not a finger stick!) for people older than 45 if they have no risk factors. Start earlier if they have risk factors such as obesity and/or a family history.

The American Association of Clinical Endocrinologists recommends starting screening at age 30 if any risk factors are present.

Abdominal Aortic Aneurysm

One-time screening for abdominal aortic aneurysms (AAAs) is recommended in men age 65–75 if they have a history of smoking (ACC/AHA and USPSTF) or in men over 60 if they had a sibling or parent with AAA (ACC/AHA). Repeat screening is not recommended. No organization recommends screening in women.

Breast Cancer

Breast cancer screening using breast self-exams, clinical breast exams, and mammography is now somewhat controversial. We discuss the topic in the Oncology section.

Prostate Cancer

Prostate Specific Antigen (PSA) testing has contributed to the increased finding and treatment of early prostate cancer. Although no trials have been concluded indicating its effectiveness as a screening test, consumer demand is making it a common lab test.

The American Urological Association and ACS recommend PSA and digital rectal exam yearly for men > 50 years old.

The ACP recommends that annual PSA be discussed with men between the ages of 50 and 69 to determine if they want it based on benefits and harms. No PSA screening is recommended for men > 70 years. In general, discuss screening at age 40 with African-Americans and in patients with a family history of early prostate cancer. The digital rectal exam, previously combined with serum PSA screening, is no longer recommended by the ACP.

To add to the confusion, the USPSTF does not recommend screening at all!

When screening is recommended, most authorities say to repeat every 4 years.

Colorectal Cancer

This is discussed in depth in the Gastroenterology section.

Cervical Cancer

Pap smears have been proven effective, but the recommended intervals between these tests vary. Most recommend starting at age 21. When there have been 3 negative results with annual exams, continue every 3 years until 60–65 years old. If previous Pap smears have been negative and the patient does not have new sexual partners, patients > 65 years old do not need further smears. You do not need to get a Pap on women who have had hysterectomies for benign disease. See the Oncology section for workup of abnormal Pap smears.

HPV testing is being integrated into screening for women over 30 years of age at some institutions because the result helps you determine what to do if Pap smear cytology returns with atypical squamous cells of undetermined significance (ASCUS). Usually, the HPV test is collected with the Pap smear, but it is saved until cytology results are available. If ASCUS is discovered, then the lab is instructed to perform the HPV test (termed "reflex testing"). Women with ASCUS and the high-risk HPV types (16, 18, 31, 33, 35, 39, 45, 51, 52, 56, 58, 59, 68, 69, 82) then go to colposcopy (instead of sending everyone with ASCUS to colpo; cuts down on unnecessary procedures). Not all institutions are doing this, although it is the most cost-effective strategy for managing ASCUS.

Lung Cancer

Screening with imaging is not recommended currently. Tobacco cessation counseling is the most effective strategy.

Vaccinations

Common adult vaccinations are discussed in the Infectious Disease section.

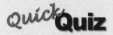

POISONINGS

OVERVIEW

The following ingestions and inhalations are those most likely to cause death in the U.S.:

- Carbon monoxide inhalation
- Overdoses of analgesics, sedatives, or antidepressants
- Ingestions of isopropyl alcohol, methanol, or ethylene glycol
- Use of illicit drugs

First, we discuss an empiric approach to overdoses; then we focus on individual ingestions. Ingestions with HAGMA and increased osmolar gaps are covered exhaustively in the Nephrology section. CO poisoning is discussed in the Pulmonary Medicine section.

OVERDOSE MANAGEMENT

General management of the obtunded or comatose patient is guided by a history, vital signs, and physical exam. Assessment of airway is most important, with immediate intubation of the patient with unstable vital signs and/or inability to protect the airway. Next, assess rhythm with an ECG and continuous cardiac monitoring and blood oxygenation with pulse oximetry.

The following interventions are usually empirically performed, except as noted:

- IV D50 if blood glucose low.
- Thiamine 100 mg IM or IV.
- ABG +/– carboxyhemoglobin level, serum basic chemistry, and general toxicology screen. Be sure to calculate the serum anion and osmolar gaps. Measure salicylate level if AG is increased.
- Serum acetaminophen level.
- Serum CPK, if patient was immobilized for long periods.
- CXR and supplemental oxygen prn.
- Naloxone IV if you suspect opiate overdose but be careful of dose (see below).

Be able to characterize the patient's physical exam and determine whether the presentation is most consistent with "excitation" or "depression" and know which ingestions are associated with the presented scenarios (Table 10-11 on next page).

In clinical practice, many patients present with coingestions, and the physical exam can be a mixed bag of signs/symptoms.

Tip: mydriasis = dilated pupils (big word, big pupils); miosis = constricted pupils (small word, small pupils).

After the patient is stabilized, consider gastric lavage with a large bore orogastric tube; this may be effective even hours after ingestion if the drug was ASA, anticholinergics, or narcotics (these cause decreased gastric motility). Lavage with only small amounts of tap water (100 cc) to prevent forcing the stomach contents into the duodenum. Follow with activated charcoal and a cathartic (sorbitol or Mg citrate). Know that activated charcoal is not effective when the overdose is with the metals lithium and iron. Continued dosing with oral charcoal is effective in decreasing the levels of a few drugs by gut dialysis (absorption via the enteric recirculation)—especially digoxin, phenobarbital, theophylline, tricyclics, and salicylates.

Note that there is a strong trend toward not lavaging patients with most overdoses. The thought is that lavage is, in most cases, ineffective; using activated charcoal with cathartics is at least as effective, if not more so.

Shock is treated with CVP monitoring, IV fluids, +/– dopamine.

Alkalinization and acidification of the serum (and hence, the urine) are based on the principle that compounds in their ionized form are less tissue-permeable and more easily eliminated by the kidneys. Weakly acidic substances ionize in an alkaline environment while weakly alkaline substances ionize in an acidic environment. Alkalinization of the urine to a pH of > 7 increases excretion of ASA, tricyclics, and phenobarbital. Acidification of the urine with ammonium chloride increases excretion of amphetamine and phencyclidine (PCP). Mix 2.75 mEq/kg in 60 cc NS and give through the gastric tube. Clamp for 1 hour. Repeat q 6 hours until urine pH < 5.0.

Important: Hemodialysis may be necessary in patients with severe overdose or renal failure. It is effective in removing drugs with low molecular weights that are not lipid-soluble, protein-bound, or tissue-bound—i.e., drugs with a small volume of distribution. These include lithium, chloral hydrate, salicylates, and alcohols (methanol and ethylene glycol). Dialysis is not effective in removing benzodiazepines, opiates, or tricyclics.

Also: Charcoal hemoperfusion (blood pumped through a charcoal filter), in contrast to dialysis, removes drugs that are lipid-soluble and protein-bound! It can also remove some of the same drugs as dialysis. Also like dialysis, it is most effective in removing drugs with a

Table 10-11: Physical Exam in Toxic Ingestions			
Physical Exam	**Category**	**Examples**
"Excited": Agitation, restlessness, hypertension, tachycardia, hyperventilation, hyperthermia, mydriasis (usually)	Anticholinergics	• Antihistamines • Neuroleptics (chlorpromazine, quetiapine) • Tricyclic antidepressants • Atropine • Antispasmodics (hyoscyamine) • Plants: Nightshade (belladonna) and jimson weed
	Sympathomimetics	• Ephedrine • Dextromethorphan (5–10x therapeutic dose) • Cocaine • Amphetamines • Methamphetamine • MDMA ("Ecstasy") • 4-bromo-2,5-dimethoxyphenethylamine ("2CB") • 2,5-dimethoxy-4-(N)-propylthiophenethylamine ("Blue Mystic")
	Hallucinogens	• Lysergic acid diethylamide (LSD) • Mescaline (peyote) • Phencyclidine (PCP, "angel dust") • Psilocybin (found in certain mushrooms)
"Depressed": Obtundation, hypotension, bradycardia, hypoventilation, hypothermia, miosis (usually)	Cholinergics	• Organophosphate and carbamate insecticides
	Sympatholytics	• Clonidine
	Opiates	• Oxycodone (frequently combined with acetaminophen; has extended-release formulations; ETH-Oxydose™, OxyContin®, OxyIR®, Roxicodone®, Percocet®) • Hydrocodone (frequently combined with acetaminophen; has extended-release formulations; Lorcet®, Lortab®, Vicodin®, Zydone®, Co-Gesic®, Hycet®, Margesic®)

low volume of distribution (V). Especially good for digoxin, theophylline, and salicylate overdoses.

SPECIFIC TOXINS

Refer to Table 10-11. Also see Table 10-12 on page 10-35 for a summary of common poisoning agents and their usual antidotes.

Anticholinergics

Don't forget the presentation of anticholinergic intoxication (discussed above and reiterated in the table). "Red as a beet; dry as a bone; hot as a hare; blind as a bat; mad as a hatter; full as a flask."

• Red: Cutaneous vasodilation
• Dry: Anhidrosis
• Hot: Hyperthermia
• Blind: Mydriasis
• Mad: Hallucinations
• Full: Urinary retention
• Antidote: Physostigmine

Acid Alcohols

Isopropyl alcohol ("rubbing alcohol") is a common solvent and disinfectant. Like ethanol, it has CNS-depressant effects. It is second to ethanol in the causes of alcohol overdose. The main metabolite is acetone, which causes a prolonged CNS effect. The acetone causes ketonuria, and the sweet odor of acetone is evident on the patient's breath. CNS depression is the major effect, although there may also be cardiac depression. Abdominal pain and vomiting are usually present. An osmolar gap of > 35 mOsm is usually seen with toxicity. Treatment: Give supportive care, including lavage if < 2 hours has passed since ingestion. Make early use of hemo/peritoneal dialysis in severe cases.

Methanol (wood alcohol) toxicity is usually due to contaminated moonshine. It is only mildly inebriating, and many signs of toxicity are delayed > 24 hours—especially visual impairment, from blurring to blindness. The toxic metabolites are formaldehyde and formic acid. Serum analysis shows an increased anion and osmolar gap. Treat with fomepizole, folic acid, and immediate dialysis. Give folic acid to increase metabolism of the formic acid.

Ethylene glycol (antifreeze). Alcohol dehydrogenase breaks down ethylene glycol to its very toxic metabolites, especially oxalate. Presence of oxalate is indicated by calcium oxalate crystals in the urine and hypocalcemia (oxalate chelates calcium). Suspect if a patient appears intoxicated but without an alcohol smell, and with a HAGMA and increased osmolar gap. Treat with

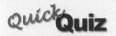

fomepizole, bicarbonate for the acidosis, calcium prn, and immediate dialysis.

Analgesics

Opiates

Think opiate overdose (especially on a Board exam) when you see the following combination of signs/symptoms: obtundation, hypoventilation (decreased rate and tidal volume), decreased bowel sounds, and constricted pupils. Know that meperidine, propoxyphene, and tramadol are associated with seizures in intoxicated patients (especially those on dialysis!); and methadone can increase the QT interval, causing *torsades*.

Naloxone is usually given IV in doses of 2 mg, up to a maximum of 10 mg. The drug should be used to reverse hypoventilation induced by opiates—it should not be used in large doses as a diagnostic tool for opiate intoxication because of the risk of inducing withdrawal in the chronic user. The dose of naloxone should be titrated to result in normal ventilation (10–14 breaths/minute), not consciousness. Too great of a dose (enough to wake someone up completely) can cause rapid reversal and withdrawal. Too small of a dose can result in a need for intubation. Chronic users of opiates, and those patients who inhaled or ingested a large dose of the drug, may require an intravenous drip of naloxone because its half-life is very short. Usually 2/3 of the dose that results in adequate ventilation is given per hour in a drip.

Know that acute lung injury is sometimes seen in opiate addicts who undergo rapid reversal of unconsciousness with naloxone + high-flow oxygen via facemask. Patients usually recover with supportive care.

Also recognize that naloxone is usually not the correct answer if a scenario presents a patient with dilated pupils.

Salicylates

Salicylates are metabolized in the liver by conjugation with glycine or glucuronide. These pathways are quickly saturated in a person who has overdosed, resulting in acidemia. The increased ASA level initially causes hyperventilation through a central effect. This has a

protective effect since the ASA crosses the blood-brain barrier (i.e., is more tissue permeable) when the system is acidemic. Acidosis can worsen if the HAGMA is compounded by lactic acidosis due to pulmonary edema. If the patient stops hyperventilating, it is probably due to respiratory muscle fatigue.

The classic presentation of the patient with an ASA overdose is tachypnea and a mixed acid-base disorder (HAGMA + respiratory alkalosis) and a history of having taken "over-the-counter" pain medicine. Depending on the dose, patients may additionally complain of tinnitus.

Treatment of salicylate overdose: Decontamination with activated charcoal with cathartic, and serum/urine alkalinization using sodium bicarbonate. Both hemodialysis and charcoal hemoperfusion have been used in severe cases (salicylate levels > 100 mg/dL). The charcoal hemoperfusion removes the salicylates better than hemodialysis but does not correct any fluid/electrolyte imbalance (patients are often hypokalemic).

Acetaminophen

90% of this drug is metabolized in the liver, by glucuronidation or sulfation, to inactive metabolites. 5% is excreted unchanged through the kidneys. The last 5% is metabolized by way of the hepatic cytochrome P-450 system to active metabolites. One of the active metabolites is N-acetyl-p-benzoquinoneimine (NAPQI), which is highly hepatotoxic. Normally, the small amount of NAPQI is quickly detoxified by reacting with the sulfhydryl group of glutathione, forming nontoxic mercapturic acid. A large overdose results in depletion of the glutathione and subsequent increase in these metabolites. A severe overdose is often followed by mild N/V/D. It is only after 24–48 hours that liver toxicity ensues.

Many intentional overdose patients present with coingestion of multiple substances. Always suspect acetaminophen as part of the clinical picture of any overdose. It is standard to check acetaminophen levels regardless of the presentation—because untreated toxicity is potentially fatal.

Alcohol-acetaminophen syndrome. Chronic moderate-to-heavy use of alcohol has a 2-fold effect: The cytochrome P-450 system is cranked up (so that more NAPQI is produced), and the amount of glutathione is decreased (so less is available for detoxifying the NAPQI). Therefore, long-time users of moderate-to-heavy amounts of alcohol who take acetaminophen in normal or higher doses are at risk for severe hepatic toxicity or liver failure.

Treatment of acetaminophen overdose: Activated charcoal is beneficial, does not hinder use of N-acetylcysteine (NAC), and is usually used if patients present within 4 hours of ingestion. Although there is great variability in the hepatic response to the overdose, a 4-hour post-ingestion acetaminophen level of > 250 µg/mL indicates a high probability of hepatotoxicity—if untreated. NAC is an effective antidote that works by increasing the availability of hepatic glutathione.

NAC is effective when given within 8 to 16 hours after the acetaminophen overdose. Even when given late in the course to a patient with significant ingestion and toxicity, it reduces mortality and improves liver function. Treatment can be initiated with either an IV or oral protocol, which varies in their duration. IV is favored if patients are vomiting or present in liver failure.

The oral NAC protocol includes a loading dose of 140 mg/kg, followed by doses q 4 hours of 70 mg/kg for 17 doses (IV uses loading of 150 mg/kg with an infusion over next 20 hours). Both protocols continue dosing until the measured acetaminophen level is undetectable or "clearly decreasing" with a minimum of dosing over 20 hours. (The specific definition of "clearly decreasing" is controversial.)

Prescription Drugs

Theophylline: This drug more often presents as inadvertent toxicity rather than intentional overdose. Toxicity often occurs in the context of the patient having been prescribed another drug (or herbal preparation) that increases theophylline levels. Suspect toxicity when you see a clinical history of obstructive lung disease and tremulousness, tachycardia/ventricular arrhythmias, vomiting, +/– seizures with a theophylline level > 20 mcg/mL. This toxicity can look like cocaine or methamphetamine use. Be aware of it in patients with asthma who also use these illicit drugs! Know the drugs that commonly interact with theophylline and increase levels: CYP3A4 inhibitors, certain macrolides, quinolones, and zileuton.

Treat with supportive care (pay attention to hypokalemia because it predisposes to ventricular arrhythmia) and multiple doses of activated charcoal with cathartic. If vomiting is too severe to allow for charcoal, give ondansetron +/– ranitidine. Treat seizures with diazepam; SVT with adenosine. Stable ventricular arrhythmias usually respond to amiodarone; treat hypotension with alpha agonists (phenylephrine or norepinephrine). Oddly, beta-blockers can reverse hypotension, if the alpha agonists don't work, but beta-blockers should be given only under the guidance of a medical toxicologist. Call poison control to get such advice. Dialysis is recommended in patients with seizures or ventricular arrhythmias.

Lithium: Mental status changes are the most common manifestation of overdose—affecting > 90%. Other CNS changes include seizures and symptoms due to encephalopathy (poor memory, incoherence, disorientation). Patients may also get parkinsonian symptoms and movement disorders. Nausea, vomiting, and diarrhea are also common. A lithium level is obtained for purposes of documenting definitive overdose, but symptoms do not correlate with levels.

Don't forget about the complications from chronic lithium use: renal tubular acidosis, nephrogenic diabetes insipidus, and sicca symptoms.

Treatment: Activated charcoal is not effective. Gastric lavage is recommended in this setting. Restore fluid and electrolyte balance, and use hemodialysis in severe lithium overdose cases. Consider severe intoxication when there are any symptoms characteristic of lithium poisoning, when the lithium levels are > 3.5 to 4 mEq/L, or when the serum level does not decrease appropriately.

Tricyclic antidepressants: These drugs are lipophilic and are protein-bound, so they have a very large volume of distribution and cannot be removed by dialysis. Clinical presentation of toxicity includes: sedation or confusion and arrhythmias.

Treatment includes gastric decontamination with activated charcoal with cathartic, if presentation is within 2 hours of ingestion. Give supportive care and monitor for cardiotoxic side effects. Tricyclics cause tachycardia and PR, QT, and QRS prolongation. The QRS prolongation is the ECG change that correlates most closely with the degree of intoxication! Ventricular tachycardia and fibrillation are also common. The cardiac problems often respond to maintaining an alkalemic state—either by hyperventilation if the patient is intubated or with IV bicarbonate. Keep serum pH 7.5 to 7.55 using sodium bicarbonate ("alkalinizing the urine"). Give lidocaine (first choice) or phenytoin as needed for arrhythmias. Use benzodiazepines for seizures.

Digoxin: This drug is not commonly prescribed, but toxicity is not uncommon because the drug has a very narrow therapeutic index. Levels do not correlate with toxicity, so you have to pay close attention to signs and symptoms. Clinical presentation of toxicity includes anorexia, N/V, belly pain, confusion, weakness, changes in color vision, scotoma, and bradycardia with hypotension. The presentation can appear as if the patient is being overtreated with an antihypertensive drug—this is important because patients who take digoxin will often also take antihypertensives. Labs may show potassium disturbances (hypo- in acute toxicity; hyper- in chronic toxicity) and acute kidney injury, which is often the cause of the increase in the serum level.

Know the commonly used drugs that can increase digoxin levels when coadministered: diltiazem, verapamil, amiodarone. Because digoxin is cleared by the kidney, decreases in GFR increase the serum level.

Treatment consists of continuous cardiac monitoring. PVCs are common. Other conduction abnormalities include AV block with junctional escapes and serious ventricular arrhythmias. The ECG should be evaluated periodically because digoxin can flatten or invert T waves, shorten the QT interval, and depress lateral ST segments (findings often referred to as "dig effect").

Treat with activated charcoal if presented within 2 hours of ingestion. Treat patients who have serious ventricular

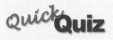

Quick Quiz

- What drugs are used to treat acetaminophen overdose?
- What ECG finding correlates most closely with the degree of intoxication of a tricyclic antidepressant?
- A 30-year-old man presents with acute MI. What drug should be ruled out as the cause?
- Memorize Table 10-12.

arrhythmias (tachycardia, fibrillation, complete heart block, Mobitz II, and symptomatic bradycardia), serum K > 5 mEq/L, and renal failure or mental status changes with Fab fragments (a digoxin antibody). Be aware that presenting hyperkalemia will rapidly reverse with Fab antibodies, so do not be overly aggressive in treating hyperkalemia.

Much controversy exists about whether to give calcium to patients with hyperkalemia from digoxin toxicity (to stabilize cardiac membranes). Conventional teaching is to withhold the calcium (and this is what we have written in our Nephrology section), but several case reports and retrospective studies show that calcium does not harm these patients. The current standard, however, is not to give calcium if you are giving Fab antibodies because the hyperkalemia is rapidly corrected, and arrhythmias are unusual.

Illicit Drugs

Cocaine: Cardiotoxicity can occur no matter what the route of use. This drug causes rhythm disturbances (including V fib/tach), ischemia (irrespective of whether the patient has preexisting atherosclerotic disease), myocarditis, and systolic dysfunction. Suspect

Table 10-12: Toxins and Antidotes	
Toxin	**Antidote(s)**
Acetaminophen	N-acetylcysteine
Digoxin	Ag-binding fragment
Opiates	Naloxone
Benzodiazepines	Flumazenil (Mazicon®)
Nitrates	Methylene blue
Iron	Deferoxamine
Carbon monoxide	Oxygen
Ethylene glycol	Fomepizole
Methanol	Fomepizole
Organophosphates	Atropine, Pralidoxime
Cyanide	Nitrates, Na-thiosulfate

use in a young patient presenting with MI. Seizures and stroke are also common with cocaine; consider it in patients with first-time seizure. Know that beta-blockers are not used in this group to treat angina or verified myocardial ischemia. Instead, nitro, calcium-channel blockers, and BDZs are 1st-line treatments.

Methamphetamine is a powerful CNS stimulant that acutely increases the release of epinephrine, norepinephrine, serotonin, and dopamine. Consider overdosage in the sweaty, severely agitated or psychotic patient with tachycardia and hypertension. Severe tooth decay occurs in chronic users. Acute treatment of the severely agitated patient is with IV benzodiazepines first and then antipsychotics, such as haloperidol, if needed. IM doses are given if unable to give IV. Watch for rhabdomyolysis in these patients by monitoring electrolytes, BUN, Cr, CPK, serum lactate, liver enzymes, and clotting times.

Phencyclidine (PCP) can cause acute psychotic agitation, seizures, dystonia (including laryngospasm), and hypertensive crisis. Severe dystonia can cause rhabdomyolysis. Treat with a calm environment and IV BDZs as needed, with supportive care for complications such as rhabdomyolysis.

Heroin is an opiate (see above). Be careful with the use of naloxone in chronic users because of the risk of precipitating withdrawal if you overshoot in dosage. Heroin intoxication is sometimes difficult to differentiate from alcohol intoxication because both substances are CNS depressants. But alcohol usually does not constrict the pupils or decrease the bowel sounds.

MDMA (3,4-methylenedioxymethamphetamine; ecstasy) is commonly used by young people in the setting of parties or raves. Use results in feelings of euphoria, loss of inhibitions, cozy feelings of intimacy, and increased sexual arousal due to an increased release of serotonin. The drug is commonly perceived as being very mild with minimal risk and physical effects; but in actuality, ecstasy possesses properties that resemble a combination of amphetamines and peyote (stimulant + hallucinogen). The drug is taken in tablet form, and overdoses can result in death.

Side effects of MDMA include bruxism (jaw grinding), anxiety, sweating, hypertension, and tachycardia. Dangerous complications include severe hyponatremia, malignant hypertension, stroke, cardiac ischemia, arrhythmias, aortic dissection, and serotonin syndrome. Hyperthermia and rhabdomyolysis are possibilities, especially in patients who dance all night and use ecstasy.

Activated charcoal is given if the patient presents within 1 hour of ingestion. In intoxicated states, most symptoms respond to benzodiazepines (hypertension, tachycardiac, agitation). Haloperidol can potentially exacerbate hyperthermia. Arrhythmias respond to calcium-channel blockers. Beta-blockers are not recommended because of the possibility of unopposed alpha-adrenergic stimulation.

Hyponatremia usually responds to water restriction; hyponatremic seizures should be treated with hypertonic saline.

LSD: Lysergic acid diethylamide is referred to as "acid" and causes hallucinations. Fatalities and morbidity during use are unusual—usually attributable to bad decisions being made while intoxicated.

Miscellaneous

Carbon monoxide: Carbon monoxide quickly binds with hemoglobin—with an affinity of ~ 250x greater than O_2. This carboxyhemoglobin (COHb) decreases arterial oxygen content, which leads to tissue hypoxia.

Symptoms are progressive and range from headache and lightheadedness to lethargy to unconsciousness to coma to death.

Be especially suspicious if the patient has been working around cars, gas/oil heating units, or generators. Typical real-life scenarios:

- Car exhaust: Garage music band using a running car to warm up the garage on a cold winter day—with the door closed.
- Exhaust from gasoline-powered generators: Especially suspect after electricity has been lost, such as after a flood, hurricane, or ice storm.
- Poor combustion in heating unit: Suspect when a patient calls from home in winter (especially near start of the cold season) and says the family is suffering from headache and lightheadedness. The patient may sound slow to respond. Or the patient calls in the winter and complains of headache and lightheadedness, which improves when he goes outside.

What to do? The answer to any scenario in which the patient calls you with suspect symptoms, especially with the above environmental factors, is to tell the patient to leave and get the family out of the house immediately, then, you send an EMS unit there.

CO poisoning is responsible for most deaths in patients with smoke inhalation, so don't forget to check COHb levels when managing smoke inhalation.

The brain and heart are especially sensitive to CO. Poisoning often causes long-term to permanent CNS impairment with cognitive deficiencies (i.e., memory and learning) and personality and movement disorders.

Fetal hemoglobin has especially high affinity for CO, so treat pregnant patients aggressively.

If you suspect carbon monoxide poisoning, get a carboxyhemoglobin level. A hand-held breath analyser can quickly rule out CO poisoning, but ethanol causes false positives.

- Mild-to-moderate CO toxicity occurs at 15–30%.
- Moderate-to-severe toxicity occurs if > 30%.

- > 50% is often fatal.

"Cherry red" coloration is rare.

Treat CO poisoning with 100% O_2—this decreases the half-life of COHb from about 5 hr to 1 hr. Hyperbaric O_2 further decreases the half-life to 30 min, but its main benefit is that it decreases the CO-induced ischemic reperfusion injury to the brain.

Hyperbaric oxygen is generally given for moderate-to-severe CO poisoning. Many centers routinely use it in all patients with a COHb level of $\geq 25\%$ and in pregnant women with a level of $\geq 20\%$. Use it for all patients presenting with either of the following:

- Loss of consciousness or any focal neuro deficit
- End-organ damage, especially acidosis

Smoke inhalation: Respiratory impairment results from the noxious chemicals in the lungs or laryngeal/airway edema. Suspect laryngeal involvement if face or airways are burned (e.g., singed nasal hairs). Don't forget about the association between CO poisoning and smoke inhalation.

Cyanide poisoning clues: Patient's breath has an almond odor and lab draw shows bright red venous blood. Cyanide immediately binds to the ferric molecule in the mitochondrial cytochrome oxidase complexes, thereby blocking cellular aerobic metabolism. These patients very quickly develop headache, tachycardia, and tachypnea. This may quickly progress to coma and various cardiac arrhythmias. Think about cyanide poisoning in patients who have been in a fire or who have received sodium nitroprusside or amygdalin (chemical derived from apricot and peach pits that is used often in herbal compounds). Laboratory evaluation routinely shows significant lactic acidosis. Diagnosis is clinical, after excluding other causes of lactic acidosis and carbon monoxide poisoning. Assays exist to find the chemical in the blood, but these are reference tests that take a long time to return.

Treatment for cyanide poisoning is the 3-step cyanide antidote package. Goal is to induce methemoglobinemia because cyanide preferentially binds methemoglobin and produces a less toxic reaction.

- **Step 1** is amyl nitrate held under the patient's nose for 30 sec.
- **Step 2** is to administer 3% sodium nitrite IV. The nitrites convert hemoglobin to methemoglobin (the ferric form of hemoglobin), which more effectively competes with the cytochrome oxidases for the cyanide. Amyl nitrate inhalation causes a 3–5% methemoglobinemia while the sodium nitrate causes 20% methemoglobinemia.
- **Step 3** is sodium thiosulfate IV, which acts as a substrate for the enzyme rhodanese. This enzyme converts the cyanide released from hemoglobin to inactive thiocyanate, which is excreted renally.

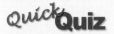

- Know carbon monoxide poisoning!
- What are the 3 drugs used to treat cyanide poisoning?
- How do you check for ongoing inorganic lead exposure? What about exposure 2 years ago? What if 10 years ago?
- What is the treatment for organophosphate poisoning?

Significant toxicity can result in a parkinsonian-type syndrome because cyanide is toxic to the basal ganglia.

Inorganic lead: There are 3 scenarios to test for lead exposure, depending on when the exposure occurred:

- For ongoing exposure, check whole blood lead level.
- After exposure has occurred, RBC protoporphyrin and zinc protoporphyrin levels will remain elevated for several months.
- For evaluating the effect of exposure from years before, the best test is to measure urine lead 24 hours after giving 1 gm of EDTA.

Organic lead is lipid-soluble and rapidly excreted, and previous exposure is not detectable!

Insecticide: Organophosphate and carbamate poisonings present identically. Symptoms include increased salivation, miosis (small pupils), N/V/D, and abdominal cramps. Affected patients also complain of chest tightness and generalized weakness. Organophosphates are more toxic than carbamates; they bind irreversibly to acetylcholinesterase, whereas the carbamate binding is reversible. This is reflected by a decrease in the level of RBC (not plasma!) acetylcholinesterase for several months after organophosphate poisoning, while it returns to normal within hours after carbamate poisoning.

Treatment for insecticide poisoning: The route into the body is dermal absorption (especially organophosphates), so decontaminate by removing clothes and showering with soap. For moderate-to-severe symptoms, give atropine (1–2 mg IV, repeat q 5 min prn). Additionally, for organophosphates only (not carbamate), give 2-protopam (2-PAM) IV.

DRUG WITHDRAWAL

So far, the discussion has focused on intoxication. You should also know the following presentations of specific drug withdrawal.

Heroin is the major opiate associated with physiologic withdrawal—it also has the most addictive potential. Symptoms usually start within 6 hours to a day after the last dose of drug—or can present immediately in the setting of opiate antagonists (e.g., naloxone, buprenorphine). Early symptoms include agitation, rhinorrhea, tearing, muscle aches, nausea, vomiting, abdominal pain, and diarrhea. Definitely think about this entity in the tearful patient who is yawning—those two activities usually don't go together.

Exam shows constricted pupils, yawning, hyperactive bowel sounds. Tachycardia and hypertension are seen in patients in severe distress (but are often not present in most patients).

Methadone is given to patients who are chronically addicted to opiates and present in acute withdrawal. If the patient desires to stop opiate use entirely because of addiction and refuses methadone, symptoms can be ameliorated with clonidine and diazepam. Promethazine is given for vomiting, and loperamide helps the diarrhea.

Benzodiazepine (BDZ) withdrawal can be fatal. It presents with anxiety and tremulousness, melancholy, and sometimes psychosis/seizures. Time of withdrawal from last dose depends on whether the drug used has a short or long half-life (up to 3 weeks for diazepam). Ideally, these drugs would be tapered over a prolonged period when a patient is discontinuing chronic use. Withdrawal is treated with long-acting benzodiazepines.

Ethanol: Patients severely addicted to ethanol start having withdrawals within about 6 hours from the last drink (and can happen even though the patient still has a measurable blood alcohol level. If it's lower than the patient is accustomed to having, then he can withdraw). Symptoms get more severe as time passes. After about 12 hours, patients usually have an isolated generalized seizure. The next phase is hallucinosis, where the patient's sensorium is intact and BP/pulse are normal; but, he sees, hears, and feels nonexistent phenomena. The last withdrawal syndrome is delirium tremens (DTs). DTs are marked by autonomic instability and delirium. Untreated, they last about 5 days. Complications include volume depletion, hypokalemia, hypomagnesemia, and hypophosphatemia. For DTs, give good supportive care, replace thiamine with glucose, and give long-acting BDZs. Replace electrolytes prn. Watch out for refeeding hypophosphatemia (discussed in the Nephrology section). For patients who can be frequently observed, give repeat BDZ doses when symptoms recur. In situations where observation is not as feasible, fixed dosing schedules are used. Do not use haloperidol for the delirium because it can precipitate seizures. Chlordiazepoxide can be given orally to patients not in DTs, if they desire to quit drinking, to prevent alcohol withdrawal.

OPHTHALMOLOGY

OVERVIEW

Aqueous humor is produced by the ciliary body, flows through the pupil into the anterior chamber, and then goes through the trabecular network and into the Schlemm canal. The greater the resistance to this flow in the trabecular network and the Schlemm canal, the greater is the intraocular pressure. Normal pressure is < 21 mmHg (Figure 10-6).

GLAUCOMA

Overview

Glaucoma is an insidious disease in which a prolonged, elevated intraocular pressure causes progressive visual field loss due to optic nerve damage. There are 4 broad classifications: primary open-angle (POAG), closed-angle, congenital, and secondary. Know the specifics about POAG and closed-angle glaucoma.

Primary Open-Angle Glaucoma

Primary open-angle glaucoma (POAG) is the most common type. It is called "open-angle" because the orb has elevated pressure with no closure of the inlet of the trabecular network. These patients suffer unnoticed gradual loss of peripheral vision that can progress to legal blindness before it is detected. Risk factors include advanced age, family history, African-American race (5x increased risk compared to other races), and increased intraocular pressure.

Be suspicious and refer for ophthalmologic evaluation those patients with risk factors and/or those who have "cupping" on funduscopic exam ("cupping" = cup occupying > 50% of the optic disc; normal cup occupies < 50%).

Screening of POAG: The American Academy of Ophthalmology recommends a comprehensive eye exam by an ophthalmologist or skilled optometrist after the age of 40. After the initial screening exam, repeat screening is usually recommended every 3–5 years in patients without risk factors and every 1–2 years for those with one or more risk factors (borderline intraocular pressure, cupping, African-American race, and

family history). Patients with DM should be seen yearly. They also recommend that African-Americans have periodic exams between the ages of 20 and 39 as well. For all individuals older than 60, a complete exam should be done every 1–2 years. The USPSTF found insufficient evidence to recommend for or against screening adults for glaucoma.

Treatment of POAG. The following meds are used:

- **Prostaglandins** (topical) are 1st-line drugs because of the once-daily dosing and the few systemic side effects, especially compared to the topical beta-blockers. These are expensive!

- **Beta-blockers** (topical): Dramatically decrease intraocular pressure—probably by decreasing production of aqueous humor. It is thought aqueous humor production is mediated by tonic sympathetic (beta) stimulation.
  - Nonselective (timolol, carteolol, levobunolol, metipranolol)—may cause lethargy, bradycardia, and exacerbations of COPD
  - Beta$_1$-selective (betaxolol)

- **Adrenergic agonists**: Decrease production of aqueous humor by constricting the vessels of the ciliary body and decreasing ultrafiltration. In chronic use, they increase aqueous humor outflow.
  - Nonselective (epinephrine)
  - Alpha$_2$-selective (apraclonidine, brimonidine)

- **Cholinergic agonists**: Stimulate parasympathetic receptors at the neuromuscular junctions → retracting the longitudinal muscle of the ciliary body → opening the trabecular network. These cause pupil constriction.
  - Direct-acting cholinergic agonist (carbachol, pilocarpine)
  - Cholinesterase inhibitor (demecarium, echothiophate, physostigmine)

- **Carbonic anhydrase inhibitors**: Convert CO_2 to bicarbonate. In the eye, the formation of bicarbonate → sodium into the eye → sodium is followed by water → which increases intraocular pressure.
  - Oral (acetazolamide; rarely causes idiosyncratic aplastic anemia)
  - Topical (brinzolamide, dorzolamide—equally effective)

Closed-Angle Glaucoma

Primary closed-angle (angle closure, narrow angle) glaucoma, the most severe form of narrow-angle glaucoma, is an ocular emergency—know it well. Risk factors include age > 40 years, female, hyperopia (farsightedness), Asian race, and family history. The elevated intraocular pressure is caused by mechanical obstruction of aqueous outflow through the trabecular network, due to an anomalous iris configuration or iris neovascularization. The resulting rapid increase in intraocular pressure causes redness, severe eye pain, nausea,

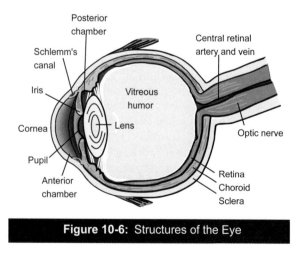

Posterior chamber
Schlemm's canal
Iris
Cornea
Pupil
Anterior chamber
Vitreous humor
Lens
Central retinal artery and vein
Optic nerve
Retina
Choroid
Sclera

Figure 10-6: Structures of the Eye

- What is the difference between open-angle and closed-angle glaucoma? Which is a medical emergency? What is the treatment for open-angle glaucoma?
- What is the treatment for closed-angle glaucoma?
- Describe the findings with retinal detachment.
- What is the treatment for retinal detachment?
- How do retinal artery occlusion and retinal vein thrombosis differ?

and halos around lights. It can also be associated with headache and present similar to migraine. Low-light conditions that precipitate pupillary dilatation (e.g., night time or in the movie theater) is associated with onset.

Physical exam shows decreased vision, increased intraocular pressure (often > 30 mmHg), a narrow anterior chamber (difficult to assess), corneal edema, conjunctival hyperemia, and a fixed, mid-dilated pupil.

Ideal treatment includes immediate ophthalmologic referral for a laser iridotomy. If an ophthalmologist cannot see the patient within an hour, institute immediate treatment with:

- Pilocarpine drops: Constricts the pupil
- Beta-blocker drops: Decreases intraocular pressure
- Alpha-agonist drops: Decreases intraocular pressure
- Oral acetazolamide

Instructions with over-the-counter medications often include admonitions to "avoid use in patients with glaucoma" (decongestants). These warnings apply only to patients with closed-angle glaucoma not already treated with iridotomy.

THE RETINA

Retinal Detachment

Retinal detachment may occur spontaneously. It often presents as flashes or streaks of light (photopsias), showers of black dots (hemorrhage), or a "shade coming down" or "waving curtain" in a portion of the visual field. Visual acuity may be normal initially. Myopia (nearsightedness) is the biggest risk factor.

Presumptive diagnosis is based mainly on history, but occasionally a portion of the retina appears elevated or folded on ophthalmoscopic exam.

Treatment: This condition requires an emergent referral because untreated partial detachment can progress over hours to total retinal detachment with permanent blindness. Small retinal detachments are treated with laser surgery to tack down the area. Larger detachments

require scleral buckling (a band around the sclera to restore contact of retina with the wall of the eye), transscleral drainage of fluid, vitrectomy (removal of vitreous), or injection of gas or other fluid into the eye (to tamponade the retina).

Retinal Vascular Occlusion

Retinal Artery Occlusion

Occlusion of the central retinal artery—usually embolic—causes sudden, painless, unilateral blindness. This is a true ocular emergency in which every minute counts. Retinal edema (sparing the relatively thin fovea) creates pallor and the appearance of a "cherry red spot" in the macula.

Treatment is directed toward dislodging the embolus and includes ocular massage, paracentesis of the anterior chamber (to lower pressure), and carbogen ($O_2 + CO_2$) inhalation to dilate retinal vessels. While waiting for the ophthalmologist, have the patient get into the Trendelenburg position and breathe into a paper sack. You may massage the affected globe with your index fingers (5 sec pressure, 5 sec no pressure, repeat). Unfortunately, all these temporary measures are rarely effective. Patients subsequently require a thorough systemic evaluation for embolic and carotid disease.

Retinal Vein Thrombosis

Retinal vein thrombosis causes sudden, painless, near-total loss of vision. Causes include hypertension, polycythemia vera, and Waldenström macroglobulinemia. Retinal edema is accompanied by hemorrhage—not a cherry red spot.

Diagnosis is made with an ophthalmoscopic exam showing a "blood and thunder" fundus with multiple hemorrhages.

Unlike retinal artery occlusion, there is no effective acute treatment, and it is not considered an emergency.

Macular Degeneration

Age-related macular degeneration is the leading cause of irreversible acquired legal blindness in developed countries. There are 2 types: atrophic (or "dry") and neovascular (or "wet"). Atrophic is the most common.

Risk factors for both types include smoking and low levels of zinc and antioxidants in the diet. However, most trials have not shown any reduced risk with vitamin supplementation or antioxidants. One recent trial, however, did show reduced risk with B vitamin supplements. This is being investigated further.

Background: The fovea is responsible for fine (20/20) visual acuity. The fovea and surrounding retina is called the macular area. Although the macula comprises only 2% of the visual field, 25% of the cone photoreceptors are here, and it correlates with 50% of the primary visual area of the brain.

Atrophic age-related macular degeneration causes a gradual loss of central acuity down to 20/400 (peripheral vision is spared). Neovascular age-related macular degeneration is somewhat amenable to treatment with laser photocoagulation and photodynamic therapy.

OPTIC NERVE

Optic Neuritis (ON)

ON is an inflammation of the optic nerve and is a frequent presentation of multiple sclerosis (MS).

ON presents with ocular pain, especially with eye movement. On exam, the optic disc is usually normal initially ("the doctor sees nothing, the patient sees nothing") and

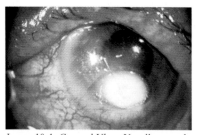

Image 10-1: Corneal Ulcer. Usually caused by improper use of contact lenses. It is especially seen with the extended-wear contact lenses.

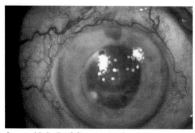

Image 10-2: Proliferative Diabetic Retinopathy. Rubeosis. Blood vessels grow onto the iris. This may cause intractable glaucoma. Also caused by central retinal vein thrombosis.

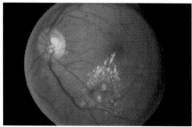

Image 10-3: Hard Exudate as seen in non-diabetic retinopathy. This is caused by leakage of protein and lipids from capillaries. Treatment is photocoagulation of the leaking capillaries.

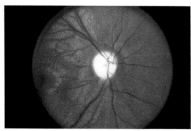

Image 10-4: Optic Atrophy has various causes, including proliferative diabetic retinopathy and central retinal artery occlusion. In older patients, also consider ischemic optic neuropathy.

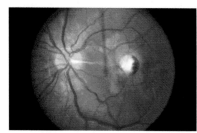

Image 10-5: Toxoplasmosis.

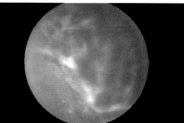

Image 10-6: Proliferative Diabetic Retinopathy. Vitreous hemorrhage.

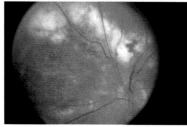

Image 10-7: CMV Retinitis. Especially seen in people with AIDS.

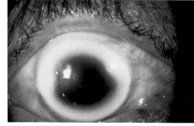

Image 10-8: Arcus Senilis. Common in older patients. In patients < 40 yrs, it may be a sign of a lipid disorder.

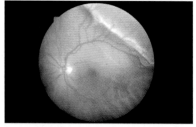

Image 10-9: Retinal Detachment. This usually occurs in very myopic people. It often occurs after a vitreous hemorrhage.

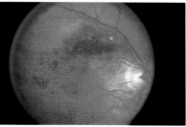

Image 10-10: Branch Retinal Vein Occlusion (BRVO). Main cause is hypertension but also seen with diabetes and with hyperviscosity syndromes. Think of this as exaggerated AV nicking with the artery pinching off the vein.

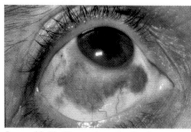

Image 10-11: Heterochromia, Ocular Melanosis. This is a normal finding in darkly pigmented persons. Rarely caused by Fuch's iridocyclitis.

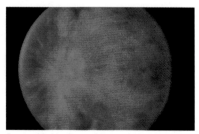

Image 10-12: Central Retinal Vein Thrombosis (CRVO). Same causes as BRVO.

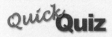

Quick Quiz

- What is the leading cause of acquired legal blindness in the U.S.?
- Optic neuritis may signal the development of what neurologic disorder?
- What is vitreous hemorrhage?

only later develops pallor. Refer the patient to an ophthalmologist. IV glucocorticoids improve vision more quickly, but these are controversial because patients not given steroids ultimately regain vision as well. Typically, an MRI is done, looking for evidence of MS.

Ischemic Optic Neuropathy

Ischemic optic neuropathy is the feared complication of giant-cell (temporal) arteritis. Other signs and symptoms are those of polymyalgia rheumatica: malaise, fever, weight loss, muscle aches, jaw claudication, elevated ESR (erythrocyte sedimentation rate). Corticosteroids are started as presumptive treatment even before the diagnostic temporal artery biopsy is done.

VITREOUS HUMOR

Vitreous degeneration occurs in all elderly persons. They tend to get bothersome floaters, brief unilateral flashing lights (from the vitreous traction on the retina), and vitreous detachment (with a sudden shower of floaters and flashing lights). Vitreous detachment is not dangerous unless it damages the retina.

Vitreous hemorrhage is a cause of sudden, painless loss of vision. It is caused by either a vitreous detachment tearing a retinal vessel or as a result of breakage of the fragile blood vessels in diabetics with the neovascularization (proliferative diabetic retinopathy).

Any patient with vitreous detachment should be referred to an ophthalmologist, who will look for current retinal detachment and also defects that, when repaired, may forestall future retinal detachment. The eye with vitreous hemorrhage must be examined by ultrasound to check for retinal detachment.

CATARACTS

The crystalline lens of the eye is a clear biconvex structure behind the iris and supported by the zonules. The lens is initially pliable and reactive to accommodation. As the lens ages, it gets less pliable and may get less clear. Any lens opacity is called a cataract. Cataracts cause a very gradual, painless, progressive loss of vision. Treatment is cataract surgery with replacement of the lens.

CRANIAL NERVE DYSFUNCTION

Suspect cranial nerve involvement in the patient who presents with sudden onset of painless double vision (Figure 10-7).

6th CN (abducens; CN VI) supplies the lateral rectus. Paralysis: Cannot move the eye laterally.

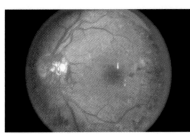

Image 10-13: Papilledema. Seen with increased intracranial pressure. Think of tumor and pseudotumor cerebri. Mimics optic neuritis/ papillitis, except papilledema is bilateral.

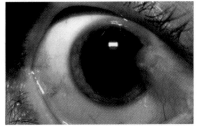

Image 10-14: Allergic Conjunctivitis. Usually seasonal.

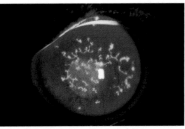

Image 10-15: Herpes Keratitis of the cornea. Frequently recurs.

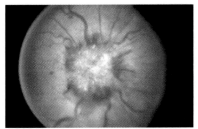

Image 10-16: Proliferative Diabetic Retinopathy with disc neoplasia.

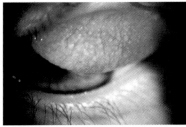

Image 10-17: Pterygium. Associated with exposure to ultraviolet light and dry wind. Seen in farmers, professional golfers, etc.

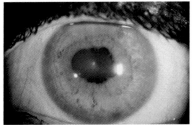

Image 10-18: Synechiae. This is a possible sequela of iritis (iridocyclitis). 90% of iritis is idiopathic, but it is seen in inflammatory diseases such as viral infections and connective tissue diseases.

4th CN (trochlear, CN IV) paralysis: Eye is deviated upward and the head tilted toward the uninvolved side (Bielschowsky sign).

3rd CN (oculomotor, CN III). Motor: Two branches, superior and inferior. The superior branch supplies the superior rectus and the levator palpebrae superioris (eyelid muscle). The inferior branch innervates the inferior rectus, inferior oblique, and the medial rectus. There is also a parasympathetic component of CN III, which is yet another branch. It results in tonic constriction of the pupil. Complete paralysis of CN III results in an eye that is deviated "down and out" (due to unopposed activity of the superior oblique [CN IV] and lateral rectus [CN VI]), a ptotic eyelid, and a dilated pupil. If the eye is not dilated, the patient probably has diabetic vascular disease affecting only the somatic branches.

EYE INJURY

Trauma

Check acuity; inspect anterior chamber for layered blood (hyphema), corneal laceration, subconjunctival hemorrhage, puncture wound, or pupil distortion; use ophthalmoscopy to confirm clear view of retina and no other signs of hemorrhage. If there is pain, instill fluorescein to check for corneal abrasion and evert, inspect, and swab the upper lid, looking for a foreign body. Any abnormal finding, except perhaps a small corneal abrasion, requires consultation.

Alkali Injury

Alkali injury is a special form of trauma where treatment delay of minutes can devastate the eye. Alkali rapidly penetrates the cornea and enters the anterior chamber, where it wreaks havoc. Treatment is immediate, consisting of profuse irrigation, with lid eversion to remove any

alkali-containing particles. Check pH of tears to confirm that it is normal before discontinuing irrigation. Vessels may be blanched by alkali solution in severe injury, paradoxically creating the appearance of a "white and quiet" eye.

RED EYE

Assessment

The most common cause of a red eye is conjunctivitis. Conjunctivitis may be bacterial, viral, or allergic. By far the most common cause of acute red eye is viral—usually adenovirus. A red eye may also indicate more urgent conditions. Workup should include evaluation of certain key differentiating features—acuity, pain, and photophobia (light sensitivity). Other features to assess are preauricular adenopathy, amount and type of discharge, and the location and amount of redness.

1) Decreased visual acuity may indicate a serious problem requiring prompt consultation. Check for an afferent pupillary defect (seen more often in serious eye conditions).

2) Photophobia is a key feature of iridocyclitis (and other more serious conditions), which should be evaluated promptly (within 24 hours) for possible intensive topical steroid treatment.

3) Type of redness. Bright red confluent blood is seen with subconjunctival hemorrhage. Ciliary flush (red near corneal limbus only in a sun ray-like pattern) suggests iridocyclitis, keratitis, or angle closure. Diffuse conjunctival hyperemia is nonspecific.

4) Pain is not common in typical infectious causes of red eye. In patients who have photophobia, foreign body sensation, and/or vision complaints, consider the more serious conditions of anterior uveitis, keratitis, or acute closed-angle glaucoma.

5) Preauricular adenopathy (may be tender) is highly suggestive of adenoviral conjunctivitis.

6) Discharge, if purulent, suggests bacterial etiology. Clear exudate more likely suggests viral. White, stringy exudate may be allergic, especially if associated with pruritus. If there is no pruritus, it is more likely dry eye (keratoconjunctivitis sicca—see below).

Anterior Uveitis

This is autoimmune inflammation of the anterior eye structures. It occurs as a solitary problem but is also seen with many diseases (e.g., spondyloarthropathies, sarcoidosis, lupus, vasculitides). You can make a presumptive diagnosis with symptoms of ocular pain, photophobia, and a ciliary flush with a normal cornea and normal intraocular pressure. Slit lamp exam reveals inflammatory cells floating in the aqueous humor or deposited on the corneal epithelium. This presentation requires emergent referral! Treatment: Steroids (reduce inflammation and scarring) and cycloplegics (to prevent synechiae).

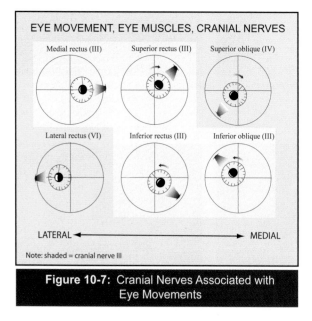

EYE MOVEMENT, EYE MUSCLES, CRANIAL NERVES

Medial rectus (III)   Superior rectus (III)   Superior oblique (IV)

Lateral rectus (VI)   Inferior rectus (III)   Inferior oblique (III)

LATERAL ← → MEDIAL

Note: shaded = cranial nerve III

Figure 10-7: Cranial Nerves Associated with Eye Movements

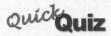

- Know the eye movements associated with the 3rd, 4th, and 6th cranial nerves.

- What virus is usually responsible for conjunctivitis?

- A contact lens wearer presents with severe keratitis and says she uses tap water frequently for lens care. What organism should you consider?

Keratoconjunctivitis Sicca (Keratitis)

This is most common in the elderly and in middle-aged women. It may be an early sign of systemic inflammatory disease, including Graves disease, rheumatoid arthritis, and sarcoidosis. Treat most cases with artificial tears (electrolyte solutions, methylcellulose, or other formulations).

Viral Conjunctivitis

Viruses are, by far, the most common cause of red eye. Patients have diffuse conjunctival hyperemia and profuse watery discharge (often with other signs/symptoms of a viral infection). No specific treatment, just practice strict hygiene. Adenovirus is one of the most common etiologies, especially in the summer around swimming pools. It should resolve in 5–7 days.

Bacterial Conjunctivitis

Bacterial conjunctivitis may be caused by staph, strep, *H. influenzae*, *Pseudomonas*, *Moraxella*, or *Neisseria*. Most cases of bacterial conjunctivitis will resolve in 5 days even without treatment; but, we do treat and follow closely because the patient can develop vision loss.

Red eye with profuse purulent discharge is the typical presentation.

Treat uncomplicated cases with topical erythromycin, sulfa, or polymyxin/trimethoprim (drops or ointment; drops are preferred for adults because vision is blurry for ~ 20 minutes after insertion). Remember: Some patients have sulfa allergy, so worsening conjunctivitis after sulfa treatment may be due to allergy. Reserve quinolones for the more serious cases.

If complicated, obtain cultures (swab conjunctiva), initiate treatment with a quinolone, and refer to an ophthalmologist. Aminoglycosides are not used much anymore because they irritate the cornea and cause inflammation after a few days.

Neisseria conjunctivitis (can be gonococcal or meningococcal) is a "hyperacute" (severe conjunctival discharge and redness) conjunctivitis that requires early recognition and aggressive topical treatment to prevent progression to corneal perforation. Systemic therapy is also indicated.

Patients who use extended-wear contact lenses have an impaired ability to fight conjunctivitis and are at high risk for developing vision-threatening complications. Always consider an ophthalmology referral at presentation if the patient wears lenses.

Pseudomonas conjunctivitis can progress to corneal perforation overnight in these patients. Any contact lens wearer with conjunctivitis should immediately discontinue use of the lenses. Start these patients on a topical quinolone to cover *Pseudomonas* and refer to an ophthalmologist if the patient doesn't improve within 24 hours.

Acanthamoeba is a known cause of infection with lens-wearers, especially if the patient uses tap water for lens cleaning. Usually it progresses rapidly to keratitis.

Infectious Keratitis

Think about bacterial keratitis in patients who wear contact lenses and who present with a painful eye that is difficult to keep open. Non-lens-wearers can also get bacterial keratitis, especially if immunosuppressed. Organisms usually responsible: Staph, *Pseudomonas*, and pneumococcus.

On exam, the eye is red with a mucoid discharge and a visible white spot (corneal opacity) that is easily seen with a penlight. Fluorescein staining shows the area as well.

Treatment includes emergent referral to an ophthalmologist.

Viral keratitis can be caused by reactivation of latent herpes simplex. It may present similarly to bacterial conjunctivitis discussed above. Fluorescein staining shows a characteristic dendritic branching pattern. Risk factors for reactivation include laser eye treatments and immunosuppression. Diagnosis is purely clinical because most patients have antibodies to HSV, and viral culture takes days. Treatment is with oral or topical antivirals (but not both). Know that topical steroids can seriously exacerbate the infection, so do not prescribe any topical steroids for an eye unless you are certain that the underlying diagnosis is not herpes keratitis. Some patients have problems with recurrent disease (similar to fever blisters from HSV); these patients can be managed with chronic oral antivirals.

OTHER EYE INFECTIONS

Endophthalmitis

Endophthalmitis (infection inside the eye) can have an ocular (traumatic) or systemic (blood stream seeding) source—and can be bacterial or fungal. The most common presentation is bacterial infection after cataract surgery, and the organism is usually a coagulase-negative *Staphylococcus*. Patients present with decreased visual acuity, hazy cornea, pain, and hypopyon (layering of white cells visible in the anterior chamber.) Refer immediately; the ophthalmologist will do vitrectomy and culture the vitreous fluid, then intraocular antibiotics are injected (vancomycin + [ceftazidime or amikacin]). Systemic antibiotics are added in severe cases, although utility is controversial. It is important to choose antibiotics that cross the blood-brain barrier; otherwise, the drugs will not reach the vitreous fluid. Cataract lenses do not have to be removed, unless the infecting organism is a fungus. Remember: If trauma to the orbit is involved, suspect *Bacillus cereus*!

Candida endophthalmitis is seen more commonly because of the widespread use of prolonged intravenous access and cases of fungemia. *Candida* can reach the eye via trauma or bloodstream infection. Bacterial and fungal endophthalmitis present similarly, which is the reason why cultures are of paramount importance in post-surgical patients. Risk factors for candidemia include long-term venous access, neutropenic immunosuppression, long-term broad-spectrum antibiotics, and corticosteroid treatment. Know that injection drug users who dilute drugs (usually heroin) in contaminated lemon juice are at increased risk. Treatment includes removal of the lens and systemic azole antifungal treatment (not ampho B because it does not achieve high levels in the eye).

Periorbital and Orbital Cellulitis

Periorbital cellulitis usually is a rapidly progressive cellulitis of the periorbital area, which may become orbital if not treated. Patients present with warmth, redness, and swelling around the eye. Key physical exam finding is normal extraocular muscle movement without diplopia or pain with eye movement.

If the patient has disconjugate gaze, diplopia, or pain with eye movement, it is probably the result of infection that has moved into the orbital space. This warrants a periorbital CT or MRI, and IV antibiotics with staph and strep coverage.

Chalazion

Chalazion is caused by obstruction of one of the tarsal (meibomian) glands forming a small nodule found in the tarsus under the eyelid. Not a problem unless secondary infection occurs. Such infections often require ophthalmologic surgery.

Stye

Stye is an abscess at the base of an eyelid. Treat it with warm compresses and a topical ophthalmologic antibiotic. Occasionally, it will require drainage.

EYE EMERGENCIES – REVIEW

Briefly, here is how to approach ophthalmologic emergencies.

Treat emergently and immediately refer:

- Alkali burn, trauma, orbital cellulitis, central retinal artery occlusion, angle-closure glaucoma, optic nerve infarction in giant-cell arteritis

Refer immediately without on-site treatment:

- Penetrating ocular injury, endophthalmitis, retinal detachment, keratitis/keratoconjunctivitis

Refer to be seen within 1–2 days:

- Retinal vein thrombosis, optic neuritis, and vitreous detachment/hemorrhage

HEARING LOSS

Hearing loss is conductive, sensorineural, or both.

CONDUCTIVE HEARING LOSS

Conductive hearing loss occurs because something blocks sound from entering the inner ear (otitis media, eustachian tube blockage, otosclerosis, TM perforation, and ceruminosis—or any other impaction of the external canal).

Otosclerosis is an autosomal dominant trait with poor penetrance. It is much more common in Caucasians than in African-Americans. 10% of Caucasians develop otosclerosis; 1% become symptomatic.

SENSORINEURAL HEARING LOSS

Sensorineural hearing loss is caused by either cochlear damage or nerve damage (CN VIII). It may be caused by viral infections, ototoxic drugs, meningitis, cochlear otosclerosis, Ménière disease, acoustic neuromas, or aging (termed "presbycusis").

Presbycusis is characterized by bilateral symmetrical sensorineural hearing loss in the frequencies > 2,000 Hz. 1/3 of persons older than 65 years have some form.

Ménière disease is uncommon. Affected patients have recurrent, severe attacks of vertigo that persist for several hours and often are associated with vomiting and prostration. Patients have tinnitus, fullness in the ear, and progressive hearing loss (which is frequently one-sided) until deaf, at which time symptoms stop!

Diagnosis is made with the combination of typical clinical symptoms and demonstration of sensorineural hearing loss on audiometry. Treatment of acute episodes is benzodiazepines and antiemetics (not meclizine!). Chronic treatment includes avoidance of caffeine and salt, with the addition of diuretics if symptoms continue.

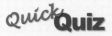

Quick Quiz

- What is the best way to diagnose an acoustic neuroma?
- A Rinne test is done. The patient can hear the tuning fork more loudly when it is on the bone. What does this mean?
- A Weber test is done on the same patient. He can hear sounds more loudly on the left side. What does this mean?

Acoustic neuromas (vestibular schwannomas) are benign, very slow-growing tumors of the eighth cranial nerve. Patients usually present with tinnitus, unilateral hearing loss, and gait imbalance. MRI is the diagnostic test of choice. Treatment is radiosurgery or surgical resection.

Acute sensorineural hearing loss should be evaluated and treated immediately. If the patient cannot be seen immediately, he should be put on prednisone (dose 40–80 mg/day) and evaluated as soon as possible.

RINNE AND WEBER TESTS

Know how to perform the Rinne and Weber tests to differentiate between conductive and sensorineural hearing loss.

Rinne test (Figure 10-8 and Table 10-13) is based on the observation that air-conducted sound is normally louder than bone conducted. The base of the vibrating 256 Hz (best) tuning fork is placed over the mastoid, and the sound of this bone-conducted hearing is compared to the air-conducted sound the patient hears when the tuning fork is placed next to the ear on the same side. With no hearing loss, the air-conducted sound is loudest. With conductive hearing loss, the bone conduction is louder. With sensorineural hearing loss, both air and bone conduction are decreased, but the air conduction is perceived as being louder.

Weber test consists of placing the base of a 256 or 512 Hz tuning fork on the middle of the forehead. The patient tells you whether the sound lateralizes to one side

or stays in the middle. If the sound is perceived as being in the middle, the patient either has normal hearing or the hearing loss is symmetrical. If the sound lateralizes, there is either a conductive hearing loss in the ipsilateral ear or sensorineural loss in the opposite ear.

You can simulate the Weber test by humming and sticking your finger in one ear (causing a conductive hearing loss). If your hearing is normal, the sound lateralizes to the plugged-up ear.

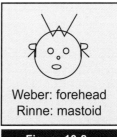
Weber: forehead
Rinne: mastoid
Figure 10-8

OFFICE PSYCHIATRY

PSYCHOSOCIAL DISORDERS

Eating Disorders

Anorexia nervosa syndrome usually begins post-puberty and in early adulthood. It almost always occurs in middle-to-upper-class Caucasian women. Anorexia may have a genetic component (concordance in monozygotic twins and increased risk in 1st degree relatives). Currently, data do not support any increased incidence of sexual abuse in anorexics.

Diagnosis is clinical. Typically, diagnosis consists of a combination of the following:

- Weight loss has resulted in a weight at least 15% under ideal.
- Patients have a preoccupation with food and have an intense fear of becoming fat.
- There are disturbances in the way body weight and size are experienced. These patients have a distorted self-image and, despite often extreme weight loss, they not only deny thinness but complain of feeling fat. This is a "soft" criterion because many young women have a similar self-perception, although without the weight loss.
- Women have had absence of 3 or more consecutive menstrual cycles.

In advanced cases, patients become emaciated, bradycardic, and hypotensive. Lab studies show anemia,

Type of Hearing Loss (examples)	Rinne Position A = Air (i.e., fork held next to ear) Position B = Bone (i.e., base on mastoid)	Weber Tuning fork base held at middle of forehead
None	Sound A > B	Sound does not lateralize
Sensorineural loss (in left ear)	Left ear: Both A & B decreased equally so still: Sound A > B	Lateralizes to the right ear
Conductive loss (in left ear)	Left ear: B > A	Lateralizes to the left ear

Table 10-13: Diagnosing Conductive vs. Sensorineural Hearing Loss with the Rinne and Weber Tests

hypokalemia, and hypoalbuminemia. These patients are at risk for sudden death from ventricular tachyarrhythmias, especially when refeeding.

Treatment. It is important to establish a supportive advisor role with the patient. Patients are very resistant to psychotherapy, and outpatient supportive care often works just as well as inpatient therapy. Explain the dangers of starvation, such as sudden death, and set realistic, short-term goals for weight gain. Acknowledge the patient's perception and continually reinforce that you will not let her get fat as she gains weight. Treatment is long-term with frequent failures and setbacks. Antidepressants may exacerbate severe anorexia because some are dietary depressants. Cyproheptadine, an appetite stimulant, may help a little. Outcome is very poor in 20–30%. Anorexics are more likely to abuse drugs and have comorbid anxiety, obsessive-compulsive, and/or personality disorders.

Bulimia is the term used for binge eating of large amounts of food, followed by purging—either with vomiting or with laxatives. It may be a variant of anorexia nervosa, and many bulimia patients have a history of anorexia in their past. Even so, these patients are usually not < 85% of ideal weight.

Diagnosis of bulimia is clinical. Typical symptoms of bulimia:

* Recurrent episodes of binge eating. At least 2 per week for at least 3 months
* Sense of lack of control over eating behavior
* Overly concerned with body weight and shape
* Regular use of self-induced vomiting, laxatives, dieting, fasting, and vigorous exercise to prevent weight gain

Physical exam may show erosive skin lesions on the fingers where the teeth cause injury during attempts to induce vomiting. Dental erosions and an increase in the size of the salivary gland are also seen. The most common lab abnormalities are hypokalemia and metabolic alkalosis from vomiting and laxative use. Think about bulimia in young women presenting with a Mallory-Weis tear or severe GERD.

Treatment is again supportive, with the focus on slowly decreasing the amount of food eaten and decreasing the frequency of binge-eating episodes. Treatment, as with anorexia, is long-term, with frequent failures and setbacks. Antidepressants may help.

Anxiety Disorders

Anxiety disorders are classified in 2 ways:

1) Generalized anxiety disorder, which is chronic and low-grade
2) Panic disorder, with brief and dramatic panic attacks

Generalized anxiety disorder. DSM-IV diagnostic criteria include: anxiety/worry about several activities or events that is more than what is reasonable for the events for ≥ 6 months. Generalized anxiety disorder is associated with substance abuse and other psychiatric diagnoses: obsessive-compulsive disorder, depression, panic disorder, and social phobias. Somatic complaints are common (fatigue, memory problems, tension, inability to sleep).

Treat with behavioral therapy. Know that several brief encouraging follow-up visits to a primary care physician has the same effect as prescribing benzodiazepines. Patients who require more than behavior therapy can be treated with SSRIs +/– benzodiazepines (BDZs). Abuse of BDZs is very low in this patient population. Buspirone is useful as a BDZ substitute. Chronic treatment is usually required.

Panic disorder is diagnosed when 4 attacks have occurred within 1 month, or 1 or more attacks are followed by 1 month of intense fear of another attack. These patients often have phobic avoidances of places or situations associated with attacks. Secondary major depression is a common complication. Treatment of panic disorder is usually with SSRIs and anxiolytics, such as benzodiazepines or buspirone HCl. The optimal treatment is an SSRI, with only short-term use of benzodiazepine. Psychotherapy may have some benefit. Longer-acting benzodiazepines (e.g., clonazepam) are preferred over alprazolam.

Bipolar Disorder

Bipolar disorder may present as solely manic or hypomanic (mild manic) episodes—the patient may never have had a depressive episode. Most manic patients are euphoric and have inflated self-esteem, decreased need for sleep, and pressured speech. Hypersexuality is common, as is overspending. Some patients are just irritable, possibly also paranoid—this is termed dysphoric mania. Psychotic symptoms are common during manic episodes. The depression is identical to common depression. Lithium, valproic acid, and carbamazepine are effective for most cases. Sometimes, antipsychotics are used in patients who have psychotic features.

The atypical antipsychotics (e.g., olanzapine) do not have the side effects associated with haloperidol; but the atypical drugs are associated with weight gain, diabetes, and hyperlipidemia. Know that many of the antiepileptic drugs are associated with increased risk of suicide. Also know that thiazide diuretics, ACE-inhibitors, and NSAIDs increase the lithium level. Refractory bipolar disorder is often treated with electroconvulsive therapy.

Depression

Depression is discussed briefly in the Geriatrics section (see page 10-15). Of course, this does not mean it occurs only in the elderly, but the general population has the same treatment options as the elderly.

- A young woman is brought in by her husband for weight loss and lack of menses for 6 months. What diagnosis should you consider?

- How does anorexia nervosa differ from bulimia?

- Describe a patient with neuroleptic malignant disorder.

Medication Complications

Neuroleptic malignant syndrome (NMS) is an idiosyncratic response to potent neuroleptics, resulting in autonomic dysfunction, extrapyramidal symptoms, and high fever. The fever may reach 106° F. The neuroleptics most commonly involved are haloperidol, piperazine phenothiazines, and thiothixene. NMS is thought to be due to a depletion of dopamine. It persists for up to 10 days after the drug is stopped. Treatment is to stop the causative drug and cool down the patient. Give oral dopamine agonists also to counteract the depletion. Bromocriptine is the drug of choice, but you may also use amantadine and dantrolene.

Serotonin syndrome. One of the functions of serotonin in the brain is to modulate body temperature. Serotonin drugs can cause derangement in thermoregulation—a condition termed "serotonin syndrome." Think about it in patients who are on at least 1 serotonin drug, but it more often occurs in patients on 2 or more serotonergic drugs. Onset is usually within 6 hours of starting the new or additional drug. Serotonin syndrome can have the presentation of SSRI overdose.

Clinical presentation is anxiety, disorientation, sweating, tachycardia, hypertension, vomiting, and diarrhea. Hyperthermia can be marked. Exam may show rigidity, hyperreflexia, and tremors. This condition looks like neuroleptic malignant syndrome, toxicity from anticholinergics, or overdose of sympathomimetics. Labs may show metabolic acidosis and evidence of rhabdomyolysis.

Treat by discontinuing the serotonergic drug and giving supportive care, including cardiac monitoring. BDZs are helpful for the anxiety and tachycardia. The syndrome usually resolves in 24 hours. The hyperthermia often results from muscle rigidity, so very hyperthermic patients usually require intubation and paralysis. Cyproheptadine is a serotonin antagonist that is given in severe cases.

GENETICS

Histocompatibility antigens are the antigens involved in graft rejection. Many of the histocompatibility genes are closely grouped on chromosome 6, and this area is called the Major Histocompatibility Complex (MHC).

The human MHC is termed HLA.

There are 3 classes of antigens found on cells that are associated with the HLA. Again, all the HLA genes are on chromosome 6.

Class I HLA antigens: All have the same molecular weight. These antigens are produced by the HLA-A, HLA-B, and HLA-C regions on chromosome 6. These antigens are on most body cells except RBCs.

Class II HLA antigens are in the HLA-D region.

Class III HLA antigens are formed in the HLA-B–D region. They consist of 3 complement component structures.

General review of transcription and translation: The DNA has coding sequences called exons, separated by non-coding sequences called introns. The gene for 1 small protein may consist of 20 of each, with 95% of the space being introns. The full gene (introns + exons) is transcribed by DNA dependent RNA polymerase into RNA. The introns are then spliced out of the RNA before it leaves the nucleus, thereby forming the messenger RNA (mRNA). The mRNA is then translated into protein: Each 3-base sequence comprises a codon, which determines the amino acid that will be attached when it is translated.

Point mutations are a change to a single base. It can result in either a missense or a nonsense mutation. Missense mutation is when a point mutation causes a different amino acid to be produced, as in SS (valine is substituted for glutamic acid). Nonsense mutation produces a stop codon, which stops the translation.

Insertion and deletion mutations: These cause a "frame shift," which causes an abnormal protein from that point to the end.

Splicing mutations result from a point mutation at the area defining the junction between the intron and the exon. This results in dysfunctional proteins. Beta thalassemias often are caused by splicing mutations.

Clues for autosomal dominant disease:

- Vertical transmission (involving several generations).
- Risk to each child of affected individual is 50%.
- Male-male transmission is observed.
- Normal parents don't transmit the trait (unless a new mutation occurs).

Clues for X-linked inheritance:

- Inheritance of trait is father to daughter—all daughters of affected males are carriers; no sons of the father are affected.
- If mother is a "carrier," she has a 50% risk of transmitting the gene to her sons, and each son with a resulting abnormal X chromosome would therefore be affected. A "carrier" mother has a 50% risk of

transmitting the gene to her daughters. If a daughter receives the abnormal X chromosome, she is usually unaffected but becomes a potential carrier to future generations.

Acquired chromosomal abnormalities: A viral gene that can transform DNA is called a viral oncogene. The human chromosomes also contain genes that are associated with malignancy, called cellular oncogenes or proto-oncogenes. These proto-oncogenes probably have something to do with embryonal development and are otherwise silent, but, with certain chromosomal rearrangement, they become active. In both Philadelphia chromosome and Burkitt's, the proto-oncogene becomes active by an acquired reciprocal translocation.

The Philadelphia (Ph1) chromosome t(9;22) was the first chromosomal abnormality found to be associated with malignancy (first found in CML). The switch causes the "c-ABL" proto-oncogene to be moved from chromosome 9 to 22.

Burkitt lymphoma and its leukemic analog, ALL (FAB type 3), have a reciprocal translocation that switches the proto-oncogene "c-MYC" on chromosome 8 to chromosome 14, 22, or 2: i.e., t(8;14), t(8;22), or t(8:2). Chromosome 14 has the heavy chain locus. The lambda light chain locus is on chromosome 22, and the kappa light chain locus is on chromosome 2.

Most leukemia and lymphoma patients have a chromosomal abnormality. Solid tumors rarely have abnormal chromosomes.

WOMEN'S HEALTH

OFFICE OBSTETRICS

The following is a compilation of everything written on pregnancy in these Core Curriculum books—plus more. This compilation makes it easier to review pregnancy as a specific topic. Because this is a very important topic, consider the entire section highlighted!

Also know Table 10-14.

◆ Gastroenterology

Esophagogastroduodenoscopy (EGD) is the option of choice for workup of many GI diseases during pregnancy to limit or preclude the use of radiation.

Endoscopic ultrasonography (EUS) is normally used in evaluating pancreatic diseases. It is also used in biliary duct disease when an ERCP would normally be used but is contraindicated (e.g., gallstone pancreatitis and pregnancy).

GE reflux disease: LES pressure is decreased by progesterone (pregnancy increases GE reflux) in addition to chocolate, smoking, and some medications, especially those with anticholinergic properties.

Crohn disease treatment with meds and their use in pregnancy.

FDA risk category B (no evidence of risk in humans):

• Metronidazole (although generally contraindicated in 1st trimester)
• Prednisone
• Sulfasalazine
• Mesalamine

Olsalazine is FDA risk category C (risk cannot be ruled out).

Constipation: The altered progesterone and estrogen levels are the probable cause of constipation in pregnancy.

Pancreatitis: Cullen sign is also seen with intraperitoneal bleeding (esp. ruptured ectopic pregnancy), and Turner sign is seen with other causes of retroperitoneal bleeding.

Unlike hepatitis A, hepatitis E carries a very high risk for fulminant hepatitis in the 3rd trimester of pregnancy—with a 20% fatality rate.

Liver disease:

1st Trimester: Hyperemesis gravidarum can cause N/V, volume depletion, and mild increase in AST and ALT.

2nd Trimester: Best time for surgery for severely symptomatic gallstone patients.

3rd Trimester:

• Remember that hepatitis E can cause fulminant hepatitis in the 3rd trimester of pregnancy—with a 20% fatality rate.
• Fatty liver of pregnancy is a very serious condition in which there is microvesicular fat deposition in the liver (as in Reye syndrome), with only modest elevation of AST/ALT/Bili. It occurs in the 3rd trimester and is associated with encephalopathy, hypoglycemia (again like Reye syndrome), preeclampsia, pancreatitis, DIC, and renal failure. Early delivery is required.
• Intrahepatic cholestasis of pregnancy causes itching and increased alk phos, bili, AST, and ALT.

◆ Pulmonary

Asthma: Budesonide is okay in pregnancy (all other steroids are category C).

Tuberculosis treatment: Do not use PZA in pregnancy because it causes birth defects.

Pregnancy is generally considered an absolute contraindication for warfarin.

◆ Cardiology

Normal findings in pregnant women:

S_3: An S_3 is normal and commonly heard in children and in persons with high cardiac output, such as pregnant women. S_3 is virtually always abnormal in non-pregnant patients > 40 years old.

Most pregnant women experience some pedal edema. Flow murmurs (and S_3 gallops) are also common, and the jugular venous pressure increases.

In pregnancy, calcium absorption and excretion is increased because the active form of vitamin D, $1,25\text{-}(OH)_2\text{-}D$ is > 2x normal.

Abnormal cardiac issues in pregnancy:

Absolute contraindications to pregnancy include pulmonary arterial hypertension and Eisenmenger syndrome. In secundum ASD, aortic stenosis, and dilated cardiomyopathy, the patient must be closely watched. In aortic stenosis and dilated cardiomyopathy, patients are usually kept at bedrest. Secundum ASD patients are usually not at risk for cardiac decompensation, unless they develop atrial fibrillation.

Atrial fibrillation: Like secundum ASD above, the initial presentation of mitral stenosis (MS) in a pregnant patient may be new-onset atrial fibrillation and pulmonary edema. The increased blood volume in pregnancy can cause a precipitous exacerbation of MS—so consider treating all pregnant MS patients with digoxin.

So remember that a pregnant patient presenting with new-onset atrial fibrillation and pulmonary edema indicates a need to rule out both mitral stenosis and secundum ASD.

A maternal rubella infection during pregnancy is a common cause of patent ductus arteriosus (PDA), supravalvular aortic stenosis, branch pulmonic stenosis ("peripheral PS"), and other congenital cardiac defects.

Aortic dissection: 3rd trimester of pregnancy, systemic hypertension, cystic medial necrosis, bicuspid aortic valve, and coarctation of the aorta are predisposing factors.

Valve surgery: Porcine valves (vs. mechanical valves) are often given to women of childbearing age to preclude the use of anticoagulants during pregnancy.

Warfarin is contraindicated in pregnancy due to its teratogenic effects. It is absolutely contraindicated in the 1st trimester; although, to be safe, most physicians do not give it at all during pregnancy.

Heparin, LMWH, digoxin, quinidine, propranolol, calcium-channel blockers, and electrical cardioversion are not contraindicated. Although heparin is not contraindicated, it does cause increased morbidity and mortality in mother and child.

In 2008, the American College of Cardiology wrote a guideline specifically looking at cardiology issues in all women. The main items to know:

- Hormone therapy should not be used as primary or secondary prevention of cardiac disease.
- Antioxidants should not be used as primary or secondary prevention of cardiac disease.
- Folic acid should not be used for prevention of cardiac disease.
- Aspirin in healthy women < age 65 years is not recommended to prevent MI (but is recommended for ≥ 65 to prevent stroke).

◆ Infectious Disease

Bacterial infections:

UTIs: *Strep agalactiae* and *E. coli*. Treat with ampicillin, cephalexin, or nitrofurantoin. Ciprofloxacin is not given to pregnant women.

Table 10-14: Most Asked-About Drugs in Pregnancy	
Dangerous (do not use)	**Relatively safe drugs**
ACE inhibitors, ARBs, nitroprusside	Clonidine, labetalol, calcium-channel blockers in trials, digoxin, verapamil, procainamide
Ciprofloxacin, doxycycline, tetracycline, metronidazole in 1st trimester, podophyllin	Sulfasalazine, beta-lactams, erythromycin, azithromycin, amphotericin B
Most aminoglycosides	Gentamicin
I^{131}, methimazole	PTU
Most antihistamines	Chlorpheniramine
Warfarin	Heparin

Listeria monocytogenes infections are associated with decreased cellular immunity syndromes like AIDS, lymphoma, and leukemia, but they are also seen in neonates, the elderly, and pregnant women. Suspect this in a pregnant woman with a UTI and negative urine culture.

Strep agalactiae (group B) is also a cause of postpartum endometritis and bacteremia. So suspect this in any woman who develops a postpartum fever!

Approximately 5% of pregnant women have *Chlamydia trachomatis* in their genital tracts; antibiotic ointment in infants' eyes at birth does not prevent this conjunctivitis (it is for GC conjunctivitis only).

Gonorrhea is more likely to disseminate in pregnant women. The newborn will be at risk for GC conjunctivitis.

Asymptomatic bacteriuria should be treated in pregnant women (1/3 go on to pyelonephritis!), neutropenic patients, diabetics, and transplant patients.

Syphilis is often asymptomatic in pregnant women.

Parasitic diseases: *Toxoplasma gondii* is serious in the immunocompetent only if acquired during pregnancy, when it can cause congenital toxoplasmosis (resulting in mental retardation and chorioretinitis). The fetus is more likely to have a congenital infection if the disease is acquired later in pregnancy (15% first trimester; 70% last trimester).

Viral infections: Viruses with the greatest teratogenic potential are CMV, varicella zoster, herpes simplex, and rubella. This is especially true if acquired in the 1st trimester.

CMV is ubiquitous and the most common cause of congenital viral infection. 1–2% of all newborns have the infection *in utero*, but only a few have any abnormalities. These abnormalities, which range from mild neurologic problems to microcephaly, usually occur in mothers with a primary CMV infection.

Rubella is German measles (ssRNA virus). If it is acquired by a pregnant patient in the 1st trimester, there is an 80% chance that the baby will have congenital defects—usually severe. Defects include cataracts, heart problems, mental retardation, and fetal death. It is diagnosed in the mother by the hemagglutination-inhibition test. If this test is negative in a newly exposed pregnant patient, repeat it in 3 weeks (after incubation period) before making any decisions. If it is then positive, a therapeutic abortion should be considered. You can diagnose rubella prenatally by finding rubella IgM antibody in fetal blood. Immune globulin will not prevent the infection, but it may give some fetal protection in the patient who declines therapeutic abortion.

Varicella-zoster infection has a slight risk of causing congenital defects. The pregnant woman with chicken pox has a 10% chance of developing severe pneumonia.

HIV: There is a mother-to-fetus transmission risk of 30%. This is reduced to < 1% with 3-drug antiretroviral therapy (ART). So ensure that all pregnant women with HIV receive ART.

◆ Nephrology

During pregnancy, there is increased calcium absorption and excretion because the $1,25\text{-}(OH)_2\text{-}D$ is $> 2x$ normal. Even so, frequency of renal stones is the same as in the non-pregnant patient. The urinary tract of the pregnant patient is dilated and, if stones do develop, most pass easily!

There are 4 categories of HTN in pregnancy:

1) Chronic HTN: Preexisting HTN or HTN before 20th week of gestation
2) Preeclampsia: HTN + proteinuria after 20th week of gestation in woman with no history of HTN
3) Preeclampsia that complicates chronic hypertension: Worsening HTN + proteinuria after 20th week of gestation in a woman with history of controlled, chronic HTN
4) Gestational HTN occurs after 20th week and has no proteinuria

The Joint National Committee (JNC) 7 report's stages of HTN do not apply in pregnancy. HTN in pregnancy is defined as mild if BP is 140–159/90–109 and severe if SBP $\geq 160/110$.

Eclampsia is defined as grand mal seizures in a woman with preeclampsia or gestational HTN.

Preeclampsia (or pregnancy-induced hypertension) more commonly occurs in primigravidas, usually in the 3rd trimester, and resolves after delivery. It is defined as [SBP > 140 or DBP > 90] and proteinuria > 300 mg in 24 hrs in a pregnant woman > 20-weeks gestation. The elevated blood pressure must be sustained with at least 2 readings at least 6 hours apart.

Preeclampsia may be symptomatic or asymptomatic (both have HTN and proteinuria). Symptoms of preeclampsia can be mild (headache, vision changes) or severe (seizures, low platelets, stroke or intracerebral hemorrhage, pulmonary edema, hepatic and/or renal failure, and placental abruption). HEELP syndrome is preeclampsia with elevated liver enzymes, low platelets, and microangiopathic hemolytic anemia.

Treat hypertension in pregnancy (regardless of category) to prevent stroke—treatment of the BP does not affect the outcome of preeclampsia (weird … but true). Know that pregnant women with hypertension are at risk for adverse fetal outcomes if blood pressure is driven too low. This is one patient group in whom we actually have higher BP goals, not lower! Each 10 mmHg reduction in SBP is associated with a reduction in fetal birthweight.

Quick **Quiz**

- A pregnant woman has a DVT. What commonly used anticoagulant is contraindicated?

- Is an S_3 gallop normal in pregnant women?

- What do you have to rule out in a pregnant patient who presents with new-onset atrial fibrillation and pulmonary edema?

- Is electrical cardioversion possible during pregnancy?

- Should asymptomatic bacteriuria in a pregnant woman be treated?

- What is the problem with rubella being acquired in the 1st trimester?

- What is the maternal-to-fetal transmission rate of HIV without ART? With ART?

- How do you make the diagnosis of preeclampsia?

- What are the symptoms that may occur with preeclampsia?

For women with preeclampsia, recommendations are to start treatment if:

1) Symptoms are present, or
2) Asymptomatic women when SBP ≥ 150 or DBP ≥ 95 (although these specific numbers are controversial), with a target BP goal of < 130–150/80–100 mmHg

Bedrest is still recommended for asymptomatic or mild preeclampsia (especially if before 34-weeks gestation), although there are no clinical trials to suggest it affects outcome. For severe, symptomatic preeclampsia, definitive treatment is delivery. Ultimately, care providers walk a fine line between delivering a baby too early to relieve preeclampsia and allowing for longer gestational development.

Women with controlled, chronic HTN (BP < 120/80) are taken off BP meds, with frequent BP and symptom monitoring. Meds are reinstituted for same BP as mentioned above for preeclampsia (SBP ≥ 150 or DBP ≥ 95), with target of < 130–150/80–100 mmHg.

Any pregnancy complicated by malignant HTN or severe, symptomatic preeclampsia is treated with parenteral antihypertensives—labetalol is the preferred drug. Hydralazine and CCBs are also sometimes used, but there are less data for these drugs. Know that the following antihypertensives are contraindicated: ACEIs/ARBs, renin inhibitors, and nitroprusside (cyanide poisoning in the baby).

Oral agents used to treat chronic, asymptomatic pre-eclampsia, gestational hypertension, and chronic hypertension in pregnancy include labetalol (other beta-blockers have less desirable effects, so labetalol is preferred), methyldopa, extended-release nifedipine, and thiazide diuretics (but watch for signs/symptoms of volume contraction).

Be aware that eclampsia can definitely occur postpartum, although rarely. A woman who presents hypertensive with generalized seizures within 12 weeks after delivery should be considered eclamptic.

SLE with lupus nephritis. If the disease has been in remission, there is a 90% chance of a successful pregnancy. If it flares up during pregnancy, however, 25% of the fetuses die, usually from the lupus anticoagulant antibody causing thrombotic events.

Pregnancy and chronic renal failure. If the creatinine is < 2 and the patient with corticotropin-releasing factor (CRF) is not hypertensive, there is not an increased risk of abortion or malformation, and there is no increase in the rate of progression of the renal disease. There is an increased risk of pregnancy-induced hypertension.

As renal failure progresses, chance of pregnancy decreases. Dialysis patients rarely become pregnant. In stable renal transplant patients, the outcome of pregnancy is usually great!

◆ Endocrinology

In reference to the serum osmostat:

The threshold set point is decreased (ADH is released at a lower osmolality) by pregnancy and pre-menses; the set point is increased by hypervolemia, acute hypertension, and corticosteroids.

Prolactin levels: Estrogen directly inhibits dopamine outflow, so elevated PRL levels can also be seen in pregnancy and in patients taking estrogen.

About 1/3 of macroadenomas will enlarge during pregnancy. If the tumor enlarges enough to cause symptoms, bromocriptine can be restarted (or surgery, if vision is threatened). Bromocriptine is almost assuredly safe in pregnancy, and cabergoline is probably also safe (less experience). But neither drug is FDA-approved for this use.

One can usually safely give I^{131} treatment to hyperthyroid patients, but it is not safe to give it to either pregnant patients or patients with severe hyperthyroidism.

Always treat pregnant hypothyroid patients and follow their TSH levels during pregnancy—because their requirements will increase (dose needs to be increased to

50% more than the pre-pregnancy dose). Failure to treat maternal hypothyroidism during pregnancy can adversely affect the baby.

Treating Graves disease in pregnancy: Surgery may be indicated in pregnancy, in patients with an associated cold nodule or relapse after radiation, and in some young patients with a large goiter.

In working up amenorrhea: Initial labs should include a pregnancy test and FSH + LH.

Pregnancy in patients with polycystic ovaries:

Treatment of PCOS first includes education about weight loss and then is dependent on the degree of hyperandrogenism and whether pregnancy is desired:

• No hirsutism and no desire for pregnancy: Prescribe medroxyprogesterone every 1–3 months to induce withdrawal bleeding and to protect the endometrium from hyperplasia.
• Hirsute and no desire for pregnancy: Prescribe combined estrogen-progesterone oral contraceptives; hirsute symptoms can also be ameliorated with depilatories/shaving; an insulin sensitizer, such as metformin or a thiazolidinedione, may also confer a very modest additional benefit on hirsutism.
• Hirsute and desires pregnancy: Induce ovulation with clomiphene with or without metformin.

Pregnancy also increases insulin resistance due to placental hormones.

Gestational diabetes:

With pregnancy, strict control even before conception is important. Maintain FPG < 100 mg/dL and A1c < 7%. Before conception, control of blood glucose reduces fetal malformation, and, during pregnancy, it reduces miscarriages, fetal anomalies/death, and newborn problems. Tight glycemic control decreases the risk of macrosomia (birth weight ≥ 9–10 lb) and shoulder dystocia in the newborn.

During pregnancy, insulin requirements increase based on gestational age of the fetus. This increased requirement is gone immediately after delivery, so anticipate a reduction in insulin dosage of at least 50% postpartum and observe the patient carefully the day after delivery.

Know that these medications commonly employed in diabetic management are contraindicated in pregnancy:

• Statins and ACEIs are category X and should be discontinued before pregnancy.
• ARBs are category C (1st trimester) and D (later trimesters).
• Many oral hypoglycemics are category C.

C = Some adverse effect on animal studies or no controlled studies in women. Use only if potential benefit outweighs potential risk to fetus.

D = Positive evidence of human fetal risk. But may be acceptable despite the risk; e.g., life-threatening illness.

X = Causes fetal abnormalities. Do not use.

◆ **Hematology-Oncology**

Fe deficiency is commonly seen in pregnant women who have had no prenatal care.

Early menarche, late menopause, and late first pregnancy are associated with breast cancer.

◆ **Neurology**

Migraine: Because of risk of inducing ischemia, do not use triptans in pregnancy.

Pseudotumor cerebri: It usually occurs in premenopausal obese women (90%) and may occur during pregnancy.

Seizures during pregnancy:

The background risk for birth defects is 2–3%. The goal of treatment during pregnancy is to control the seizures—uncontrolled seizures can cause placental abruption and early labor and premature delivery. When the risk of teratogenicity is compared to the problems that seizures cause during pregnancy, the risk of uncontrolled seizures is greater!

Maintain a pregnant woman on monotherapy and at the lowest dose of medication possible; risk of malformations increases as each drug is added.

There is no "safe" antiepileptic drug (AED), but valproate is more likely to cause neural tube defects than other commonly used antiepileptics.

The teratogenic risk of AEDs is decreased by folic acid, and all women of childbearing age on antiepileptic drugs should take 1–2 mg of folate daily.

Physicians generally give prophylactic vitamin K during the last month of pregnancy in patients on AEDs. This is based on reports indicating increased bleed in patients on AEDs. Most recent guidelines (AAN AES 2009) say there is not enough evidence to recommend for or against use of prophylactic vitamin K.

Carpal tunnel (CTS): Know that pregnancy can cause an acute presentation of CTS that typically improves after delivery. Splints are the best treatment for this patient group.

◆ **Rheumatology**

In reference to the use of methotrexate:

Pre-existing renal or liver disease (e.g., HBV, HCV, alcohol abuse) and pregnancy are definite contraindications.

Quick Quiz

- A pregnant woman has Graves disease. What can you do to treat her?
- What is a common finding in pregnant women who have not had prenatal care?
- True or False? Dysfunctional uterine bleeding (DUB) usually does not require any workup.

Leflunomide use: Contraindicated in pregnancy.

Pregnancy and menstruation are predisposing factors to disseminated gonorrhea.

SLE and pregnancy:

SSA (Ro)/SSB (La) antibodies are associated with neonatal lupus and congenital heart block. General internists need to know about this risk when counseling women with lupus about pregnancy.

Lupus patients have a higher incidence of failed pregnancies. Risk of pregnancy complications (flare or fetal problems) is much greater if disease is active (especially renal manifestations) or if the mother has anti-ds-DNA or antiphospholipid antibodies (APS). Pregnant women with APS and a history of recurrent miscarriages can be treated with heparins (low-molecular-weight or unfractionated) plus low-dose aspirin—to decrease incidence of miscarriage. Heart block starting in the 3rd trimester can be seen in babies of mothers with SLE who have SSA (Ro)/SSB (La) antibodies.

If a SLE patient wishes to become pregnant and has had a recent lupus flare, continue the glucocorticoids. Measure baseline complements, anti-ds-DNA, SSA/SSB, and a 24-hour urine protein before or very early in the pregnancy. Flares during pregnancy are managed with corticosteroids. Refer pregnant women with systemic lupus to a high-risk obstetrician (and pediatric cardiologist, if appropriate).

Avascular necrosis of the hip: Other causes include sickle cell disease, pregnancy, HIV/AIDS, Gaucher disease, and hypercoagulable states.

◆ **Dermatology**

In reference to treatment of acne:

Comedonal (noninflammatory) acne: Topical retinoids are drugs of choice for comedonal acne. These include adapalene, tretinoin, and tazarotene. Tazarotene [Tazorac®] is contraindicated in pregnancy (category X), and topical tretinoin has been associated with fetal defects (category C)! Recommended agents include oral/topical erythromycin, topical clindamycin or azelaic acid. Topical benzoyl peroxide is also category C.

◆ **Allergy and Immunology**

Persistent nasal congestion may accompany pregnancy (rhinitis of pregnancy).

OFFICE GYNECOLOGY

Office gynecology has been partially covered in previous sections. Especially review gynecologic infections in the Infectious Disease section. Pap smear, ovarian cancer, and breast cancer are covered in the Oncology section. Osteoporosis is discussed earlier in this section. Amenorrhea is discussed in the Endocrinology section.

Know that reflex HPV testing for ASCUS is not appropriate for adolescents because they have a high rate of HPV but low rate of cervical cancer. ASCUS in adolescents should be managed with a follow-up Pap at 12 months. If they have ASCUS again at 1-year follow-up, you can still observe for another year. ASCUS x 2 years in an adolescent, however, then gets referred for colpo.

A woman should undergo endometrial assessment if she has postmenopausal bleeding:

- In the absence of HRT therapy
- After she has been on combined HRT continuously for 1 year without bleeding
- At an unexpected time during cyclic replacement

Treatment recommendations for menopausal symptoms:

Vasomotor instability (hot flashes): Short-term estrogen therapy (if no history of breast cancer or cardiovascular disease).

Urogenital atrophy: Vaginal estrogen for moderate-to-severe symptoms; moisturizers and lubricants for mild symptoms.

Dysfunctional uterine bleeding (DUB) refers to excessive bleeding due to persistent anovulation in a reproductive-age woman with ovaries capable of producing estrogen. The patient's periods may be too frequent, too long, or with too heavy of a flow. DUB is a diagnosis of exclusion. There are many causes, including hypothyroidism, liver disease, renal disease, coagulopathies, pregnancy complications, anatomic lesions, and drugs, among others.

Treatment for young women with DUB is usually oral estrogen/progestin preparations. Oral contraceptives containing 35–50 µg of ethinyl estradiol are often used. 4 tablets a day are given initially; this increases bleeding for 1–2 days and generally stops the bleeding in 3–4 days. The patient is then given 2 pills per day for 20 more days. Withdrawal bleeding will then occur within 2–5 days after ending treatment. This hormonal therapy is given for 2–3 more cycles, using 1 pill per day, and then stopped.

Premenstrual tension syndrome (PMS) is a group of symptoms, which most often start during the late luteal phase and are gone within 1–2 days of the onset of menses. The biochemistry of this dysfunction has not been established. No single treatment has been proven effective, but the cause may be multifactorial, so there are many avenues of treatment to explore with each patient. You can achieve ovulatory suppression with oral contraceptives. These patients may also respond well to the newer mini pill, which contains only progestin. Other similar options include Depo-Provera® and Norplant®. Oral natural progesterone has been used with varying success. Various dietary changes help some patients, such as avoiding caffeine, salt, sugar, alcohol, and/or chocolate. Vitamin supplements, such as vitamin B_6 and vitamin E, have also been effective for some. Magnesium 360 mg (as magnesium pyrrolidone carboxylic acid) orally tid, given from day 15 to the first day of menses, may also help. Note that no one of the above treatments is effective for everyone.

MedStudy®

IM INTERNAL MEDICINE REVIEW
CORE CURRICULUM

14th EDITION

Authored by Robert A. Hannaman, MD
with Candace Mitchell, MD

NEUROLOGY

Many thanks to Neurology Advisor:

David Lichter, MD, FRACP
Professor of Clinical Neurology
State University of New York at Buffalo
Department of Neurology
VA Western New York Healthcare System
Buffalo, NY

Table of Contents
Neurology

COMA

OVERVIEW

Lethargy, stupor, obtundation, and coma are terms that apply to diminished levels of consciousness. Consciousness depends on the degree of a person's alertness and attention. Both the reticular activating system (RAS) and the cerebral cortex must be working effectively in order to sustain normal consciousness.

So coma can be caused by either a decrease in the activity of the reticular activating system (RAS) or a process that involves the cerebral cortex of both hemispheres. The RAS resides within the brainstem, so injury to the brainstem, such as a hemorrhage in the pons or midbrain, can cause coma. Certain drugs (prescribed, OTC, and illicit) also affect the RAS directly.

Plum and Posner classify the causes of coma as any of the following:

- Supratentorial
- Infratentorial
- Metabolic
- Diffuse
- Multifactorial

WORKUP OF COMA

Neurologic Exam Findings

A thorough neurological exam is required in establishing the diagnosis and possible cause of coma. Components of the neurological examination must include observations about respiration (and respiratory patterns), pupils, and motor responses (or a lack thereof).

Motor responses, such as decerebrate and decorticate posturing, may help to localize the site of injury:

- Decerebrate posturing or rigidity occurs when the tonic labyrinthine reflex that resists gravitational force acts without modulation of the higher brain, causing extension of all extremities. This is not seen much because it indicates an effective severing of the brain from the spinal cord at the midbrain or cortex level—usually a rapidly fatal situation.
- Decorticate posturing or rigidity is caused by bleeding into the internal capsule, causing upper motor neuron damage. The resultant posturing is flexion of upper limbs with extension of lower limbs.

Respirations:

Cheyne-Stokes respiration describes a particular pattern of breathing, in which the patient has periods of hyperventilation alternating with apnea. This pattern occurs in bilateral cerebral disease, impending herniation, and brainstem lesions; it can also be due to metabolic causes.

Apneustic breathing consists of inspiratory pauses and is due to a lesion of the pons.

Ataxic breathing is very irregular and usually indicates a lesion of the medulla.

Pupils: (Table 11-1). Remember that in the comatose patient, any asymmetry between the sizes of the pupils must be considered pathologic.

Oculocephalic testing (doll's eyes) and ice-water calorics (eyes look toward the cold) test the same vestibular-brainstem-ocular muscle pathway.

Doll's eyes: If the patient is unconscious yet neurologically intact, and the head is turned, the eyes keep "looking" in the initial direction (meaning eyes don't follow the direction of the head).

The presence of doll's eyes is good; it means your patient's brainstem is intact. Absent doll's eyes is bad. If the comatose patient has neither doll's eyes nor reactive ice-water calorics, there is a problem in the midbrain or pons. Generally, doll's eyes are preserved in early metabolic coma. The exceptions are metabolic comas due to barbiturates and phenytoin.

Testing of doll's eyes, which requires moving the head, should be done only after C-spine injury has been ruled out.

Table 11-1: Pupil Size in Coma				
Size		**Description**	**Cause**	**Examples**
●	•	One dilated unreactive pupil	Parasympathetic nerve problem	Oculomotor nerve compression from uncal herniation, rupture of an internal carotid artery aneurysm
·	●	One pinpoint pupil (miosis)	Sympathetic nerve problem (Horner)	Lateral medullary syndrome, hypothalamus injury
•	•	Two midpoint nonreactive pupils	Parasympathetic and sympathetic nerve destruction	Midbrain disruption (can affect one or both pupils), anoxia, hypothermia, anticholinergics, severe barbiturate overdose
●	●	Two dilated unreactive pupils		Anoxia, hypothermia, anticholinergics, severe barbiturate overdose
·	·	Two pinpoint reactive pupils		Opiates, pontine destruction

Scans and Lab Work for Coma

Quickly obtain a CT or MRI of the brain in order to narrow the differential, especially when the cause is unclear.

CBC, electrolytes, BUN, creatinine, glucose, ABG, and toxicology screen for illicit drugs may be needed.

Other tests, such as an EEG, may be helpful to identify nonconvulsive status epilepticus, especially when there is a prior history of seizures. In one series of comatose patients in whom the cause was unknown, 8% were found by EEG to be in nonconvulsive status epilepticus.

Finally, you may need to do cerebrospinal fluid examination (including the usual bacterial and viral tests) when you suspect meningitis or encephalitis.

Evaluation of Findings

Supratentorial coma is due to an injury of the hemisphere(s). There are 2 mechanisms:

1) Lateral (uncal) herniation: An expanding mass lesion (tumor, stroke, hemorrhage) will force the uncus under the tentorium. This puts pressure on the brainstem and therefore, the RAS. Because of the course of the third cranial nerve, the herniating uncus compresses this nerve, causing an enlarged pupil ipsilateral to the supratentorial lesion.

2) Central herniation: Injury to the thalamus (such as hemorrhage) results in diminished consciousness very early in its course. Later, the pupils become mid-position and fixed. As the herniation continues, the course begins to merge with that of uncal herniation. In other words, central and uncal herniation syndromes can be differentiated early on, but their courses later merge.

Infratentorial coma is due to an injury that causes destruction or compression of the brainstem. Signs of infratentorial herniation include bilateral reactive pinpoint pupils (due to pontine involvement) and respiratory abnormalities, including cluster breathing, apneusis (deep gasping), and ataxic breathing. There are 3 possible causes:

1) Basilar artery occlusion with pontine infarction
2) Cerebellar infarction or hemorrhage
3) Posterior fossa neoplasms

Expansion of the contents of the posterior fossa force the contents of this compartment in one of two directions: up (upward herniation) or down (downward herniation). Upward herniation pushes the posterior fossa contents up under the tentorium, compressing the brainstem. Downward herniation forces the cerebellar tonsils down through the foramen magnum, compressing the medulla.

Metabolic coma. There are many, many causes of metabolic coma, including ischemia, hypoxia, hypoglycemia, organ disease (lung, liver, kidney), and drugs, among others. Patients have changes in respiratory pattern and mentation early in metabolic encephalopathy. The pupils are typically reactive until the terminal stages. Exceptions include anticholinergic toxicity, which causes fixed dilated pupils, and severe barbiturate intoxication. In addition, both hypothermia and anoxia or ischemia may cause fixed pupils of varying size. Anoxic fixed papillary dilatation lasting more than a few minutes implies severe and usually irreversible brain damage, although exceptions have been reported.

CONDITIONS THAT MIMIC COMA

LOCKED-IN SYNDROME

Locked-in syndrome is rare and is due to a lesion that involves the lower brainstem, usually the pons. Usually the cause is stroke. The RAS is spared, but almost all motor pathways from the cerebral cortex to the body are interrupted. Persons are awake and aware of the surrounding environment but may have only the ability to control eye movements. Typically, they can only communicate by using vertical eye movements (the efferent abducens nerve fibers controlling horizontal eye movements are usually destroyed), and eye blinks. Because the cerebral cortex is spared, an EEG is normal. Some patients can recover some function, so treatment should be multidisciplinary and include physical and speech therapy, pulmonary rehab, and swallowing help.

VEGETATIVE STATE

Vegetative state results from severe, bilateral cerebral dysfunction, often following a period of coma. Comatose patients who enter into vegetative states either recover or progress to death—usually within 2 weeks. The remaining vegetative patients who do not recover after 3 months are unlikely to recover. Death usually occurs within 5 years from pneumonia, urosepsis, or sudden death.

These patients typically have normal sleep-wake cycles but no discernible cognitive function. Vegetative state is often caused by anoxic brain damage; e.g., after MI. Neuropathology shows cortical laminar necrosis, which is often extensive, with a relative or complete sparing of brainstem structures (including the RAS).

BRAIN DEATH

Diagnosis of brain death requires documentation that the patient is unresponsive and lacks all brain stem reflexes, including lack of oculocephalic response to cold (ice-water) caloric testing and lack of respiratory drive on apnea testing (must be off ventilator long enough for $PaCO_2$ to rise to > 60 mmHg following 10–20 minute ventilation with 100% oxygen). EEG is helpful if it establishes there is no activity in the cerebral cortex, but it is not required for diagnosis.

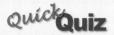

Quick Quiz

- How do you differentiate decorticate from decerebrate posturing? Which has a worse prognosis?
- What pupil finding in a comatose patient makes you think of uncal herniation?
- Where is the lesion that causes locked-in syndrome?
- Which type of migraine causes focal neurologic defects? Which type can cause incoordination?

HEADACHE

OVERVIEW

The history and examination are crucial in diagnosing the type of headache. These include the quality of pain (dull, sharp, throbbing, and constant), location, duration, exacerbating or ameliorating factors, and associated symptoms, if any.

MIGRAINE

Presentation

Migraines are unilateral (up to 60% of the time) but not consistently on the same side (unlike vascular headache secondary to arteriovenous malformation), throbbing, and last several hours. Rarely, they may last up to 3 days. Triggers include emotional stress, certain foods (e.g., chocolate, aged cheese, and other foods that are rich in tyramine), alcohol (particularly red wine or port), menstruation, exposure to glare or other strong sensory stimuli (including perfumes), and rapid changes in barometric pressure. Loud noises or bright lights (photophobia and phonophobia) may make the headache worse. Sleep and darkness may help to lessen the pain. They are frequently associated with nausea and vomiting.

Common migraine occurs without an aura.

Classic migraine (1/3 of migraines) is preceded by an aura—most commonly visual symptoms, such as sparkling lights (scintillating scotomata) or jagged zigzag lines (fortification spectra) that move slowly across the visual fields for several minutes and may leave scotomatous defects.

Complicated migraine (rare) is associated with focal neurologic symptoms, including numbness and tingling of the lips, face, and hand (on one or both sides), arm or leg weakness, slight confusion, or dizziness. In any given patient, only a few of these phenomena are present, and they tend to be stereotyped with each attack. If symptoms spread from one part of the body to another or evolve over time, they do so relatively slowly, over

several minutes (not seconds, as in seizures). Such symptoms last 5 to 15 minutes on average and are followed by unilateral headache.

Basilar migraine affects the brainstem and causes symptoms that may include vertigo, dysarthria, staggering, incoordination of the limbs, diplopia, and exceptionally, transient quadriplegia or loss of consciousness.

Acephalic migraine (migraine without headache) may present with abnormal transient neurologic dysfunction such as visual symptoms, focal sensory deficits, transient aphasia, or hemiparesis. This type frequently occurs with advancing age in patients who previously experienced common or classic migraine.

Acute Treatment of Migraine

Acute treatment refers to any treatment that is given within the first hour of the headache. Acetaminophen, aspirin, and NSAIDs are effective in some patients. If you've tried these and they've failed, then try the "triptans": sumatriptan (Imitrex®), zolmitriptan (Zomig®), rizatriptan (Maxalt®), naratriptan (Amerge®), almotriptan (Axert®), eletriptan (Relpax®), and frovatriptan (Frova®).

No head-to-head trials exist comparing the triptans, so which to choose is based on a few features of the drugs:

- Rizatriptan works fastest. But know that concomitant use of propranolol requires that you adjust the rizatriptan dose downward (propranolol increases the levels).
- Sumatriptan comes in the most dosage forms (injection, intranasal, and oral tablet).
- Combination tablet of sumatriptan + naproxen works better than either agent alone (and better than taking either agent separately but at the same time).

Because of risk of inducing ischemia, do not use triptans for any of the following conditions:

- To treat complicated or basilar migraines
- In patients with coronary heart disease or Prinzmetal angina
- In patients with history of stroke
- If blood pressure is uncontrolled
- In pregnancy

Also, do not combine triptans with monoamine oxidase inhibitors or use within 24 hours of ergot drugs.

Dihydroergotamine (DHE) may be effective in some patients. You may try narcotics, but their use should be restricted to 2 days per week. Increased use of any medication, including triptans and NSAIDs, to treat frequent headaches can incite a rebound called "medication overuse headaches." Patients should be instructed not to take analgesics more than 10 days per month. If they need meds this often, then prescribe prophylactic treatment.

Prophylactic Treatment of Migraine

These medications are taken daily. The goal of treatment is to lessen the pain and reduce the number of attacks. The frequency of attacks determines whether prophylaxis is needed: Usually, the threshold is more than 2–3 headaches per month. There is usually a lag of 2–4 weeks between the start of prophylaxis and its effect. The major categories of these agents are as follows:

- β-blockers (propranolol and timolol are FDA-approved for migraine, but atenolol, metoprolol, and nadolol are also used; be careful in patients older than 60 years and/or smokers)
- Tricyclic antidepressants (amitriptyline; side effects = oversedation, dry mouth, palpitations, orthostasis, blurry vision, weight gain, constipation)
- Tetracyclic antidepressants. These are serotonin receptor blockers (mirtazapine, venlafaxine) also known as noradrenergic and specific serotonergic antidepressants (NaSSA)
- Not enough data for SSRIs
- Anticonvulsants (valproate, topiramate; gabapentin sometimes used off-label)
- Calcium-channel blockers (verapamil, nimodipine; may develop tolerance)
- ACE inhibitors and ARBs (lisinopril and candesartan)
- NSAIDs

Definitely use prophylactic agents to treat complicated and basilar migraines.

Relaxation techniques are also helpful for patients to prevent headaches.

CLUSTER HEADACHE

Cluster headache is a distinct syndrome that frequently responds to treatment with oxygen. The term "cluster" is derived from the periodicity of the headaches: They can occur up to several times per day for a few weeks before remitting. The daily attacks may occur at the same hour each day (in 50% of patients). The pain is unilateral, severe (described as an "ice-pick" or "hot poker") and is peri- or retro-orbital. It peaks quickly in 5–10 minutes and resolves in an hour or two. In about 50%, these headaches predictably occur within 2 hours of falling asleep.

These headaches are associated with ipsilateral lacrimation, eye redness, and nasal congestion—features which help differentiate the headache from a migraine.

Cluster patients also tend to be restless during attacks, as opposed to most migraine sufferers who prefer a dark, quiet room and stillness. 70% of patients find that alcohol triggers their headache. Men are affected much more than women (4:1).

Treatment: The best acute treatment is oxygen. Inhalation of oxygen at 6 L/min x 15 minutes is usually rapidly abortive, acting to inhibit neuronal activation in the trigeminocervical complex. Triptans, including the intranasal spray, may also be effective (but are not used in patients with risk factors for heart disease and stroke). For patients who don't get better with O_2 and can't take triptans, octreotide, intranasal lidocaine, and ergot drugs are options.

Once a patient experiences the first of what will become a cluster headache, prophylactic treatment can be instituted. Verapamil is the drug of choice. Others sometimes used include lithium, methylsergide, prednisone, and topiramate. The corticosteroids are used as acute drugs while waiting for verapamil to work. Taper off the meds once the cluster is over. In refractory cases, deep-brain stimulation of the hypothalamus and greater occipital nerve stimulators have been tried in experimental settings.

TENSION HEADACHE

Tension headache is a term that is still used to describe a chronic, bilateral, constant, non-throbbing, "squeezing" type of pain, devoid of migrainous or cluster features. It may be intermittent or chronic.

Aspirin, acetaminophen, or NSAIDs can be used for acute attacks.

Preventive medication should be considered when attacks occur more than 2 days per week—this should help prevent medication overuse, which may predispose to chronic headache. Limiting treatment to 9 days per month (2 doses of meds/day) helps prevent this complication. Effective prophylactic drugs include amitriptyline and other tricyclics, tetracyclics (serotonin receptor blockers [mirtazapine, venlafaxine—see migraine prophylaxis above]), and gabapentin. Not SSRIs. Relaxation, biofeedback, and behavioral therapy are helpful in dealing with the tension that brings about the headaches.

COITAL HEADACHE

Coital headache occurs more often in men than women (4:1 ratio). The headache begins during intercourse, usually close to orgasm. It has an abrupt onset and usually resolves after a few minutes. They are benign.

If the headache does not resolve after 2 hours or is accompanied by neck stiffness, vomiting, and/or neuro deficits, consider subarachnoid hemorrhage.

POST-TRAUMATIC HEADACHE

Post-traumatic or post-concussion headache: This may occur even after a minor head injury. It may be vascular, like migraine; but, some have proposed that the headache is due to abnormal neurotransmission within the brain. Symptomatic treatment is usually effective, and the headache often spontaneously remits.

Quick Quiz

- List prophylactic treatment agents for migraine.
- Describe the common symptoms of cluster headache. How do you treat it?
- Describe the common symptoms of tension headache. How do you treat an acute attack?
- What drugs are associated with development of IIH?
- What symptoms occur in patients with IIH? What physical findings?

TEMPORAL ARTERITIS

Temporal arteritis usually occurs in patients > 55 years old. History is usually recent onset of headache. Jaw claudication, weight loss, and low-grade fever may be associated symptoms. Up to 50% of patients have a history of polymyalgia rheumatica. Do not miss this diagnosis! If untreated, irreversible vision loss is likely. Physical exam is sometimes significant for temporal artery tenderness. The erythrocyte sedimentation rate is usually very elevated. Do a temporal artery biopsy if the diagnosis is suspected. More in the Rheumatology section.

IDIOPATHIC INTRACRANIAL HYPERTENSION / PSEUDOTUMOR CEREBRI

Idiopathic intracranial hypertension (IIH; also called pseudotumor cerebri) is a set of signs and symptoms caused by increased intracranial pressure—headaches, papilledema, and loss of vision. It usually occurs in premenopausal obese women (90%) and may occur during pregnancy. It more rarely occurs in children or in men.

Obesity is strongly correlated (90–95% of patients) and causal; with the increasing obesity of the U.S. population, the incidence of IIH is also increasing.

Drugs that are associated with IIH include vitamin A (especially in the form of isotretinoin, used for the treatment of severe acne), tetracycline, and corticosteroids; but the condition may also be precipitated by steroid withdrawal.

Severe, irreversible vision loss is the major morbidity. It occurs in more than 6% of patients and is twice as common in men as in women.

Symptoms of IIH include morning headaches made worse with coughing or straining, and pulse-synchronous tinnitus. There is almost always a peripheral visual field loss accompanied by increased blind spots, which are often asymptomatic. Diplopia may result from 6th nerve paresis, and transient visual obscurations may occur.

On exam, papilledema is a hallmark finding. 6th nerve palsy may be obvious either unilaterally or bilaterally. CT/MRI is typically normal, with absence of deformity, displacement, or obstruction of the ventricular system—but may show "slit-like" ventricles. The CSF pressure is elevated, usually in the range of 250 to 450 mm H_2O (normal CSF pressure is generally < 200 mm H_2O).

Treatment of IIH. Patients are put on a low-sodium, weight-reducing diet. Drugs of choice for IIH are any of the following:

- Carbonic anhydrase inhibitors with loop diuretics
- Loop diuretics alone
- Prednisone

Prednisone works acutely but isn't recommended for chronic cases because of side effects, not the least of which is increasing intracranial pressure. Serial lumbar punctures or lumboperitoneal shunts are reserved for progressive cases refractory to medications. Unilateral optic nerve sheath fenestration may preserve vision in the acute setting.

THALAMIC PAIN SYNDROME

This causes refractory unilateral pain, which may affect the trunk, as well as the arm and leg, following weeks to years after a thalamic infarct (with hemisensory loss).

DEMENTIA

DEFINITION

Dementia is a progressive deterioration of cognitive function, sufficient to cause functional disability, in a patient with a normal level of consciousness. (Encephalopathy, on the other hand, causes altered states of consciousness—from delirium to stupor). This topic is also discussed in the General Internal Medicine section under Geriatrics.

Demented patients have deterioration in memory and other cognitive domains, including language, visuospatial skills, executive functions (including initiative and cognitive flexibility), abstract thinking, and judgment.

INITIAL WORKUP

In the initial workup, the following are causes of possibly reversible or treatable dementias that must be excluded:

- Drug-related cognitive impairment (rule this out first!)
- Vitamin B_{12} deficiency, which can also cause a polyneuropathy and myelopathy
- Heavy metal poisoning (arsenic, mercury, and lead)
- Hypothyroidism
- Chronic subdural hematomas (consider especially in alcoholics, those on anticoagulants, and elderly patients with a history of falls)

- Normal pressure hydrocephalus
- Tumors, especially involving the frontal lobes
- Also consider infection and inflammation:
  ○ HIV   ○ Chronic meningitis
  ○ Syphilis   ○ Lupus cerebritis
  ○ Sarcoidosis   ○ Vasculitis

CAUSES OF DEMENTIA

Normal Pressure Hydrocephalus

Normal pressure hydrocephalus (NPH) is a potentially treatable cause of dementia. It is characterized radiologically by enlargement of the ventricles without obstruction of the aqueduct (i.e., a "communicating hydrocephalus") and with no cortical atrophy, which might indicate hydrocephalus "ex vacuo."

NPH often occurs after head trauma, meningitis, or subarachnoid hemorrhage—and a history of one of these premorbid conditions appears to be the best predictor of a beneficial response to shunting (see below). One thought about how this develops is that there is obstruction of the outflow of cerebrospinal fluid at the level of the arachnoid granulations. However, the intracranial pressure is normal, there is no papilledema, and the person has no headache. NPH causes a gradually worsening dementia, gait ataxia/apraxia (a "magnetic" gait, with the feet apparently glued to the floor), and urinary incontinence. Often, the gait problems and incontinence precede the dementia.

The differential diagnosis of NPH includes Binswanger disease (subcortical arteriosclerotic leukoencephalopathy), which causes ventricular dilation as a result of ischemic demyelination and small lacunar infarcts in the periventricular white matter. This is common in patients with small vessel disease due to hypertension or diabetes mellitus and presents with the same clinical triad.

The treatment is lumboperitoneal shunt, and certain tests may help to identify patients who are most likely to respond to shunting. These include clinical response to LP, isotope cysternography, and dynamic MRI, which measures the direction of CSF flow (but none of these is universally reliable).

Alzheimer Disease

Alzheimer disease is the most common cause of dementia after age 60. 1st degree relatives have a 4x normal increased risk of developing it. Initial signs usually reflect hippocampal dysfunction, with poor immediate recall and short-term memory. Impairment of naming may also be an early sign. As the disease progresses, visuospatial

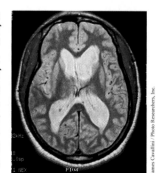

Image 11-1: Alzheimer disease; cerebral atrophy

dysfunction (including difficulty with directions and geographic disorientation), due to parietal lobe involvement, and executive dysfunction (including difficulty initiating and completing tasks, reduced spontaneity, and apathy), due to frontal dysfunction, typically appear (Image 11-1). Alzheimer disease is the prototypical "cortical" (as opposed to subcortical) dementia, and, reflecting this pathology, patients may eventually exhibit language dysfunction (aphasia), difficulty generating skilled movements (apraxia), and difficulty with object recognition (agnosia). Patients with Alzheimer's have a normal LP.

First-line treatment for Alzheimer's is the cholinesterase inhibitors (CIs):

- Donepezil (Aricept®)
- Tacrine (Cognex®; can cause liver toxicity)
- Rivastigmine (Exelon®)
- Galantamine (Razadyne®)

Best results with CIs are achieved in mild-moderate Alzheimer dementia, but other causes of dementia (e.g., multi-infarct and Lewy body dementia) sometimes also improve. CIs do not help patients with Huntington disease, however.

CIs can be combined with memantine (Namenda®), which is an N-methyl-d-aspartate receptor antagonist.

CIs provide a small benefit and help patients to carry out their ADLs (activities of daily living). Data is conflicting on their long-term effects. Not every patient receives benefit. The main side effects are anorexia, nausea, and occasionally diarrhea or bradycardia (cholinergic symptoms). Rivastigmine is available as a patch that has fewer GI side effects and is useful in demented patients who will not swallow medications. The combination of cholinesterase inhibitor plus memantine appears to be better than CI alone, especially in advanced dementia.

In an elderly patient presenting with dementia without a movement disorder, the main diagnoses to consider are Alzheimer disease, multi-infarct dementia, and mixed dementia (with both neurodegenerative and vascular components).

Multi-Infarct Dementia

Multi-infarct dementias usually have prominent motor, reflex, visual, and gait abnormalities, but they typically do not have the difficulty in naming of objects, as associated with Alzheimer disease. Another difference is the clinical course of symptoms. Multi-infarct dementia has an abrupt onset with stepwise deterioration of mental function, with more prominent fluctuations of cognition. By contrast, Alzheimer's has a slow, steady progression.

Frontotemporal Dementia

Frontotemporal dementia (FTD; previously Pick disease) is quite similar in presentation and course to

Quick Quiz

- How does normal pressure hydrocephalus present?
- How does Alzheimer's dementia present?
- How does multiple infarct dementia present?
- Dementia with predominantly psychotic features in a young person should make you suspect what infectious disease?

Alzheimer disease, but it is characterized by a more rapid and significant change in personality and behavior, often with disinhibition, language deficits, or both. The age of onset averages 58 years in FTD (relatively young, compared to Alzheimer's). The naming of FTD subtypes is evolving based on their primary manifestations; e.g., behavioral variant vs. progressive nonfluent vs. semantic. Patients with FTD have more focal atrophy of the frontal and temporal lobes on CT or MRI scan, compared with the diffuse atrophy of Alzheimer's. However, histology is the only sure way to differentiate between the two, usually at autopsy.

Currently, there are no primary pharmacologic treatments for the frontotemporal dementias. Trazodone has been shown to result in some behavioral improvement, mainly in irritability, agitation, depressive symptoms, and eating disturbances.

Creutzfeldt-Jacob Disease

Creutzfeldt-Jacob disease (CJD) is one of the very rare (1 per million people) prion diseases. It's mainly an infectious illness, but you should know that CJD is divided into sporadic (sCJD, most common, 95%), familial (about 5%), iatrogenic (iCJD), and variant (vCJD), based on observations of causes. Usually, sCJD presents around ages 55–65, and we have no idea what causes it. When you see CJD in younger patients, think either iCJD or vCJD. vCJD is believed (but not definitively proven) to be caused by the prion that causes "mad cow disease" (bovine spongiform encephalopathy) in cattle. It appears that the prion jumped species and now infects humans. iCJD is caused by receipt of infected human tissues/hormones (growth hormone, gonadotropins, dural grafts, corneal or liver transplants) or exposure to contaminated surgical instruments. Familial CJD has genetic associations, but those are not relevant for General Medicine Boards.

Regardless of cause, CJD develops as a rapidly progressive dementia (weeks as opposed to years) with characteristic startle myoclonus (response to loud noises or startle). Younger patients with vCJD tend to have dementia with predominantly psychotic features. The disease involves the cerebral cortex, basal ganglia, and spinal cord.

The diagnostic gold standard is brain biopsy. Supportive studies include: T1/T2 MRI with diffusion weighted images and Flair sequences (helps also to differentiate sCJD from vCJD), EEG (characteristic pattern of "periodic sharp waves complexes" on a diffusely slowed background), 14-3-3 protein in an otherwise bland CSF (only the National Prion Disease Pathological Surveillance Lab does this test, at Case Western, and sensitivity/specificity is < 80%). Disease is fatal in less than 1 year in > 90%.

Parkinson Disease Dementia (PDD)

Parkinson disease (PD) is caused by a loss of dopaminergic neurons in the substantia nigra. Approximately 30% of patients develop dementia in the latter stages of Parkinson's (see the later discussion under Movement Disorders on page 11-32).

Neuropathology shows Lewy bodies mixed with amyloid plaques and neurofibrillary tangles characteristic of Alzheimer disease (Image 11-2). Lewy bodies are spherical eosinophilic inclusions within the neuron (Image 11-3).

The Lewy body elements seem to correlate most with the degree of dementia, so Parkinson disease dementia is frequently called "dementia with Lewy Bodies" (DLB). DLB sometimes occurs without preceding Parkinson disease—but is otherwise the identical disease. (Some even make the distinction that PDD is what occurs in well-established PD while DLB occurs without preceding PD.)

The core clinical features of PDD/DLB (besides dementia) are spontaneous motor features of parkinsonism; recurrent, vivid, visual hallucinations (usually paranoid persecutions); and prominent fluctuations of attention and cognition.

Both the dementia and psychosis may be at least partially responsive to acetylcholinesterase inhibitors and memantine.

Typical antipsychotic drugs (e.g., haloperidol) should not be used to treat psychosis in these patients because a dramatic clinical decline may occur. However, the atypical neuroleptics clozapine and quetiapine

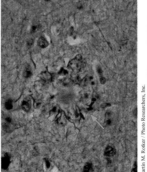
Image 11-2: Senile plaques with amyloid core

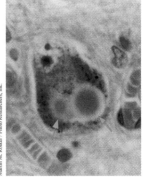
Image 11-3: Parkinson disease with Lewy bodies

fumarate (Seroquel®) are sometimes helpful and are safe if monitored appropriately.

Progressive Supranuclear Palsy

Progressive supranuclear palsy (PSP) may initially appear very similar to Parkinson disease (discussed on page 11-32), but tremor is less severe, balance is markedly disturbed earlier in the course, and there is a progressive loss of voluntary eye movements, usually starting with impairment of downgaze. Cognitive slowing (bradyphrenia) and dementia are prominent features.

Buzz words for PSP: Dementia with gaze palsy and falls.

Huntington Disease

Huntington disease causes both a dementia and a movement disorder (see other movement disorders starting on page 11-34).

The Huntington gene is on chromosome 4p, which codes for a mutant huntingtin protein that is probably toxic (the protein is spelled with an "i," while the disease is spelled with an "o"). It is inherited in an autosomal dominant fashion with complete penetrance.

This disease causes dementia, chorea, and psychiatric disturbances, including personality changes, depression, and psychosis, all of which typically begin in persons in their late 30s. Chorea is usually the heralding symptom.

Atrophy of the caudate nuclei on CT or MRI ("boxcar" ventricles) is characteristic.

Although some of the symptoms can be ameliorated with antipsychotics (neuroleptics), benzodiazepines (e.g., clonazepam), and antidepressants, there is no known treatment for the disease itself, which is invariably fatal. Genetic counseling is important for at-risk individuals.

AIDS

AIDS is the most common cause of dementia in younger patients. Dementia affects half of all AIDS patients not on antiretroviral therapy (ART). The manifestations can be mild (minor cognitive-motor disorder) to severe (HIV-associated dementia). Impairment is related to the degree and duration of immunosuppression. Controlling the virus in a patient who has had AIDS for a prolonged period, with a low CD4 count, often does not reverse dementia.

HIV/AIDS dementia is associated with cognitive impairment, movement disorders, and depression. It starts with small comprehension problems and anhedonia, accompanied by tremor and gait abnormalities. Over time, patients develop slower movements with substantial cognitive impairment. Exclude opportunistic infections of the CNS as part of the workup.

Treatment includes treating the HIV with ART, focusing specifically on designing a regimen of medications that enter the CNS at higher levels (although this has not been shown to cause neurologic improvement). Associated depression should also be treated. More on treatment of AIDS in the Infectious Disease section.

More on HIV-associated dementia on page 11-13.

Depression

Some patients with major depression present with significant cognitive dysfunction, known as depressive "pseudo-dementia." One differentiating feature is that frontal lobe release signs, such as grasp, suck, rooting, and palmomental reflexes, are common in patients with dementia, particularly if moderate or advanced, but they are not seen in isolated depression. In addition, immediate recall is usually poor in depression, due to attentional dysfunction, but good in dementia.

Depression can be reactive or endogenous. Symptoms are the same for both. In endogenous depression, patients may have an abnormal response to the dexamethasone suppression test in which the cortisol is initially suppressed as expected, but the duration of suppression is shortened (normal is > 24 hours).

DIZZINESS

SIGNS AND SYMPTOMS

When the term "dizziness" is used, one should try to differentiate among the following:

- Vertigo = a sense of spinning or swaying.
- Lightheadedness = presyncope ("I feel like I'm going to pass out.").
- Imbalance = unsteadiness.
- Vague = not one of the 3 above. It may be hard for the affected person to describe.

Nystagmus is an involuntary oscillation of the eyes. The movements may be pendular (like a pendulum) or jerk. Jerk nystagmus has 2 components: fast and slow. The eyes "drift" (= slow component), and try to quickly recover (= fast component). The type of nystagmus may indicate its cause. For instance, drugs (like antiepileptic medications) may cause horizontal and vertical gaze-evoked nystagmus (it occurs when the person looks right, left, or up)—in other words, it is present "in all directions." Isolated vertical gaze-evoked nystagmus usually indicates disease in the posterior fossa.

Jerk nystagmus is most common in vestibular disorders, but does not indicate whether the lesion is within the central nervous system, or whether it involves the cranial nerve itself. Upbeating jerk nystagmus usually indicates a lesion in the pons but can be seen in lesions of the medulla or cerebellum. Downbeating jerk nystagmus indicates a lesion at the cervicomedullary junction.

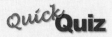

- What is the most common cause of dementia in younger adults?
- How can you differentiate dementia from depression?
- Name the maneuvers frequently employed to treat BPV.
- How does vestibular neuritis present? How long does it last?
- How does the hearing loss in vestibular neuritis differ from that in acute labyrinthitis?
- What types of TIAs can cause vertigo?

CAUSES OF DIZZINESS

Benign Positional Vertigo

Benign positional vertigo (BPV) describes recurrent, brief episodes of vertigo that are brought on by the motion of changing head position.

It is thought to be due to loose otoconia in the semicircular canal. Otoconia are crystals that reside in the saccule and utricle. When they escape this region, they may set up eddy currents in the endolymph causing symptoms of vertigo. BPV may also be caused by head trauma, labyrinthitis, or aging.

Most BPV resolves spontaneously over a couple of weeks or can be treated successfully with various repositioning maneuvers that move the otoconia to a position of the inner ear less likely to induce vertigo. These are the Epley and Semont maneuvers and their variations.

Meclizine doesn't cure BPV, but it is sometimes used to control nausea. BPV (and other causes of vertigo) is discussed thoroughly in the General Internal Medicine section.

Vestibular Neuritis

Vestibular neuritis (vestibular neuronitis, acute peripheral vestibulopathy) causes a sudden onset of non-positional vertigo that is self-limited but may last weeks to months and occasionally can recur. Vestibular neuritis is caused by an inflammatory process affecting the vestibular portion of the 8th cranial nerve and can be associated with viral infections. Tinnitus is usually absent, and hearing is not affected. Treatment is symptomatic only. When hearing loss is present, it is called "labyrinthitis."

Aminoglycoside Toxicity

Aminoglycoside toxicity can cause some initial sensorineural hearing loss and, later, intermittent mild vertigo.

Ménière Disease

Ménière disease begins in the 3rd and 4th decade of life. The characteristic triad is episodic vertigo (often associated with nausea and vomiting), tinnitus (ringing in the ears), and low-frequency hearing loss. It usually begins unilaterally but can become bilateral in 20–30% of patients. One possible cause is an increase in the endolymphatic fluid pressure, which is in part related to salt intake.

Exclude neurosyphilis as a cause of hearing loss by checking a serum VDRL or RPR.

Treatment includes dietary modification of salt, caffeine, and tobacco. If spells persist, thiazide diuretics may help. 95% of patients get their disease under control and function normally. For medically recalcitrant Ménière disease, endolymphatic sac surgery, surgical labyrinthectomy, and vestibular nerve sections remain therapeutic options.

Vertebrobasilar TIAs

Vertebrobasilar TIAs (transient ischemic attacks) may cause intermittent, recurrent vertigo. A TIA is usually easy to diagnose because it also causes other symptoms of vertebrobasilar insufficiency, such as bilateral vision loss, diplopia, dysarthria, ataxia, and bilateral extremity motor or sensory dysfunction. Workup of the posterior circulation requires special imaging. Know that the standard workup looking at only the anterior circulation (echo, carotid Doppler, and CT head) does not catch stenoses in the posterior circulation. Order Doppler of the posterior circulation or CT or MR angiography that looks at these vessels.

Know the causes of tinnitus mentioned above. Other causes include aspirin overdose and high noise levels.

SEIZURES

OVERVIEW

Partial vs. Generalized

Seizures arise from the cerebral cortex.

Postictal altered mental status is very common after a seizure—this is the main symptom used to differentiate between seizure and syncope.

All seizures can be conceptualized as either partial or generalized. The terms are used to describe the onset of the seizure. Partial (or focal) seizures begin in a part of one hemisphere, whereas primary generalized seizures begin in both hemispheres simultaneously. Partial seizures are further divided into simple partial (consciousness is maintained) and complex partial (consciousness is impaired). A simple partial seizure may evolve into a complex partial, and either type of partial seizure may evolve secondarily into a generalized seizure.

Partial seizures are more commonly due to focal brain lesions while primary generalized seizures are more commonly genetic (although there are many exceptions to this rule of thumb).

Types of Seizures

The discussion here addresses 4 main types of seizure:

1) A **generalized tonic-clonic** seizure is also known as a grand mal in older epilepsy literature. These involve both hemispheres, with resulting bilateral motor involvement. Consciousness is impaired with a pronounced postictal period. Another commonly used term to describe this type of seizure is "convulsion."

2) **Absence** seizures used to be called petit mal. These are generalized seizures with no aura or postictal symptoms. They can be induced by hyperventilating. Absences have a characteristic 3-per-second spike and wave pattern on EEG. 2/3 of affected children outgrow absence seizures.

3) **Simple partial** seizures are focal seizures that affect a small volume of cortex. Consciousness is preserved. The symptoms of a simple partial seizure depend on the region of cortex from which the event is generated. For instance, a partial seizure arising in the occipital lobe (visual cortex) may be manifested by complex visual hallucinations; e.g., spinning colorful spheres. Jacksonian seizures are simple partial seizures that involve the motor strip.

4) **Complex partial** seizures involve a large enough volume of cortex to cause a disruption in cognition or awareness. They often originate in the temporal or frontal lobes.

Pure temporal lobe seizures have no clonic motor component; patients present only with abnormal behavior or mental function.

Seizures are additionally classified as clinical, subtle, or subclinical, depending on the outward manifestation of the seizure.

Triggers for seizures in susceptible people include: alcohol, cocaine, intense emotions, strobe lighting, loud music, stress, menstruation, and lack of sleep.

SEIZURE MANAGEMENT

History

When obtaining the history, check for alcohol or drug use, head injury, sleep deprivation, diabetic history, and thyroid or parathyroid surgery.

Scans and Lab

Lab tests should include glucose, sodium, calcium, magnesium, LFTs, and BUN. If there are any meningeal symptoms, do a lumbar puncture and include a VDRL on the CSF studies.

Table 11-2: Notable Advantages and Disadvantages of Traditional Anticonvulsants		
Drug	**Used to Treat**	**Notable Advantages/Disadvantages**
Phenytoin	Partial (1) Generalized tonic-clonic (alternative)	Good: Long half-life so dose 1–2x/d. Bad: Gum hyperplasia, hirsutism, coarsening of features, lymphadenopathy, osteomalacia. Saturation kinetics so toxicity may present at near-normal doses.
Carbamazepine	Partial (1) Generalized tonic-clonic (alternative)	Good: First-order kinetics with toxicity level significantly above therapeutic range. Bad: Hyponatremia, leukopenia, thrombocytopenia, aplastic anemia, and hepatotoxicity.
Valproic acid	Generalized tonic-clonic (1) Absence (alternative) Partial (alternative, esp if it generalizes)	Bad: GI side effects (less with Depakote® formulation). May rarely cause bone marrow suppression and hepatotoxicity/liver failure.
Ethosuximide	Absence (1) only	Bad: May cause bone marrow suppression (rare).
Lamotrigine	Partial (adjunctive use)	Bad: May cause severe rash and Stevens-Johnson syndrome.
Gabapentin	Partial (adjunctive use)	Good: The only one with no significant drug interactions. Renal clearance so it is useful in those with liver disease. Bad: Ataxia, amnesia.
Clonazepam	Absence (short-term adjunctive use only)	Bad: Loses efficacy.
Phenobarbital	Partial (last choice)	Bad: Sedation in adults, hyperactivity in children, among other cognitive changes.
Note: (1) = primary drug. Note: Any of the above can cause ataxia, dizziness, and somnolence.		

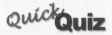

- What type of seizure is usually caused by a focal brain lesion—partial or generalized?

- In which seizure type is consciousness usually preserved?

- Name some environmental triggers for seizures in susceptible people.

- What is the treatment of status epilepticus?

- Which AEDs decrease the effectiveness of oral contraceptives?

Do either an MRI with gadolinium or a CT with contrast after the first seizure to exclude a structural abnormality; MRI is almost always the best neuroimaging test. Neuroimaging is normal in classic childhood absence seizures and certain genetic epilepsy syndromes.

An EEG showing epileptiform spikes (+/– following a slow wave) confirms the diagnosis of seizure and may localize the origin of the seizures. A normal EEG never excludes the diagnosis of epilepsy.

After an initial seizure, the risk of recurrence is increased when there is an abnormal EEG, when there is a history of a prior neurologic injury, when there is a family history of seizures, when the first seizure is a partial seizure, and/or when the MRI reveals an abnormality.

Acute Treatment of Seizures

Acute treatment of seizures: Intravenous benzodiazepines (diazepam, lorazepam, midazolam) are the drugs of choice. Phenytoin also is effective, but it takes longer to infuse.

Alcohol withdrawal seizures are usually treated acutely with IV benzodiazepines or phenytoin (again, benzodiazepines first).

Status epilepticus is defined as a seizure lasting > 30 minutes or a series of 2 or more seizures without regaining consciousness in between. It is considered a medical emergency. A cause can be determined about 2/3 of the time. Usual causes in adults include stroke, alcohol or other drugs, stopping or changing seizure medications, hypoxia, CNS infection, metabolic causes, tumor, and trauma.

Typical treatment of status epilepticus in the adult: Give thiamine and then D_{50} 50 mL if the rapid glucose test is low; then benzodiazepine (lorazepam preferred x 2 doses) followed by a loading dose of phenytoin or equivalent fosphenytoin.

Fosphenytoin lacks the injection site necrosis and cardiac rhythm complications of intravenous phenytoin infusion but is much more expensive and may result in lower initial brain phenytoin levels, based on the time required for conversion from fosphenytoin to phenytoin. Nevertheless, it is popular in the Emergency Department. If the patient is still seizing, give a 3rd dose of lorazepam, maximize the phenytoin dose, and then proceed to a barbiturate (phenobarbital or pentobarbital). ICU settings are generally needed if seizures are not controlled by the first 2 doses of lorazepam and a dose of phenytoin.

Chronic Treatment of Seizures

Antiepileptic medications are the mainstay of treatment, with monotherapy the preferred goal (Table 11-2). The choice of antiepileptic drug depends primarily on the seizure type, with additional considerations including cost, side-effect profile, and patient preference for a dosage schedule. Usually, drugs are not started until a patient has suffered at least 2 seizures.

Partial seizures: Almost all available antiepileptic drugs (AEDs) are effective in the treatment of partial seizures. The notable exception is ethosuximide, an agent that is used only to treat absence seizures. With few exceptions, the AEDs are considered equally effective. The main differences are that the older AEDs are generally cheaper; however, the newer ones are generally better tolerated with fewer side effects.

Generalized seizures: The list of effective agents for generalized seizures is shorter, and includes:

- Valproate
- Lamotrigine
- Topiramate
- Levetiracetam
- Felbamate
- Rufinamide
- Zonisamide

When can you stop the medication? This must be individualized. Risk factors include a seizure within the last 2 years, epileptiform spikes on the EEG, abnormal MRI, and a late age of onset of the seizures.

Know also that certain AEDs reduce the efficacy of oral contraceptive pills:

- Phenytoin
- Phenobarbital
- Carbamazepine
- Felbamate
- Topiramate
- Oxcarbazepine

Women taking these AEDs should use an alternate method of birth control other than oral contraceptives. Note that oral contraceptives can increase the drug concentration of the AED lamotrigine.

Options for intractable epilepsy include resective surgery (best for temporal lobe epilepsy), vagus nerve stimulation (doesn't work as well as surgery), and the ketogenic diet (works well in children).

Driving restrictions vary from state to state and continue to evolve. The Epilepsy Foundation has updated info for your state: www.epilepsyfoundation.org.

NEUROLOGY

Treatment of Seizures During Pregnancy

Know!

The background risk for birth defects is 2–3%. The goal of treatment during pregnancy is to control the seizures—uncontrolled seizures can cause placental abruption and early labor and premature delivery. When the risk of teratogenicity is compared to the problems that seizures cause during pregnancy, the risks of uncontrolled seizures is greater!

Maintain a pregnant woman on monotherapy and at the lowest dose of medication possible; risk of malformations increases as each drug is added.

There is no "safe" AED, but valproate is more likely to cause neural tube defects than other commonly used antiepileptics.

The teratogenic risk of AEDs is decreased by folic acid, and all women of childbearing age on antiepileptic drugs should take 1–2 mg of folate daily.

Physicians generally give prophylactic vitamin K during the last month of pregnancy in patients on AEDs. This is based on reports indicating increased bleed in patients on AEDs. Most recent guidelines say there is not enough evidence to recommend for or against use of prophylactic vitamin K.

INFECTIONS

BACTERIAL CNS INFECTIONS

Acute Meningitis

Diagnose with analysis of the cerebrospinal fluid (CSF). If there are focal neurologic signs or papilledema, do a CT before the lumbar puncture (LP). CSF latex agglutination tests are no longer recommended in the initial evaluation of meningitis; they test for *H. influenzae, Streptococcus pneumoniae, Neisseria meningitides, E. coli* and *Streptococcus agalactiae*. With suspected meningitis, start antibiotics immediately after the LP and blood cultures; do not wait for any LP results. Also, if doing the LP is going to be delayed more than 30–60 min, go ahead and give antibiotics immediately (before the LP)! Treatment is covered in the Infectious Disease section.

Neurosyphilis also is discussed in the Infectious Disease section.

Brain Abscess

The classic triad of symptoms is headache, fever, and focal neurological deficit(s). Most abscesses arise from intracranial extension of cranial infections (sinuses, teeth) or after skull fracture or neurosurgical procedures. Much less often, they are due to bacteremic seeding. In adults, the most common organisms are staph and strep species (e.g., *S. epidermidis* after a penetrating head injury), but don't forget about *Nocardia*. In the immunocompromised, consider toxoplasmosis.

VIRAL CNS INFECTIONS

CSF in Viral Encephalitis

With viral encephalitis, CSF has increased lymphocytes, normal to slightly increased protein, and normal glucose. EEG is almost always abnormal with diffuse slowing or focal temporal changes. The MRI is more sensitive than CT and may show hemorrhagic changes.

Herpes Simplex Encephalitis

Herpes simplex encephalitis is the most common type of non-epidemic viral encephalitis. In adults, it is usually due to a reactivation of the HSV-1 virus, although 25% are due to primary HSV-1 infection. HSV-2 is sexually transmitted and can cause aseptic meningitis during primary infection. HSV-2 less commonly causes encephalitis.

Varicella zoster virus (VZV) can also cause encephalitis, especially in the immunocompromised; and, it is associated with vesicular lesions that can be confused for herpes simplex. It's important to think about VZV because the dose of acyclovir required to treat is higher.

Treat herpes encephalitis with IV acyclovir and assume it is caused by VZV until you can exclude (so, use higher initial doses of acyclovir). Much more on herpes in the ID section.

Mosquito-Borne Arboviruses

If mosquitoes are around, think about arboviruses, especially eastern/western equine and St. Louis encephalitis viruses. West Nile virus tends to cause encephalitis only in the aged with comorbidities and in the immunocompromised (causes "West Nile fever" in younger and healthy patients).

Diagnosis of Viral Encephalitis

Polymerase chain reaction (PCR) DNA amplification of the herpes viruses now allows for an easy, rapid, and accurate diagnosis of herpes simplex and zoster.

Acute and convalescent serum titers are drawn to diagnose most arboviruses.

West Nile diagnosis requires finding antibody in spinal fluid.

Viral culture of spinal fluid is useful to identify most other causes of simple viral meningitis/encephalitis.

Viral Myelitis

Myelitis is infection of the spinal cord—a classic viral cause is poliomyelitis! Usually this presents as "transverse myelitis," meaning it affects a transverse segment of the cord. Common causes today are other enteroviruses (coxsackie and enterovirus) and flaviviruses, such as West Nile. Other forms of myelitis (less segmental) can be caused by herpes simplex, varicella zoster, and Epstein-Barr.

Quick Quiz

- What AED is most likely to cause neural tube defects?
- What are the typical CSF findings in viral encephalitis?
- How does treatment of CNS varicella differ from CNS herpes simplex?
- What is the cause of PML?

Slow Viruses and Prions

Slow viruses:

- Subacute sclerosing panencephalitis (SSPE) is caused by the measles virus; most cases occur around age 10, many years after the initial infection.
- Progressive multifocal leukoencephalopathy (PML): See below and also under Demyelinating Diseases on page 11-30.

Prion: Creutzfeldt-Jacob disease (CJD): See under Dementia, which starts on page 11-5.

HIV

Infection with HIV can result in dysfunction of any part of the nervous system. Patients get subacute encephalitis, peripheral neuropathies, vacuolar myelopathy, and aseptic meningitis.

HIV-associated cognitive impairment is common. It ranges from asymptomatic to mild to what is called HIV-associated dementia (HAD).

Know that the differential diagnoses include progressive multifocal leukoencephalopathy (below), toxoplasmosis (below), and lymphomas.

Since the use of ART, the incidence (new cases per year) of HIV associated dementia in the U.S. has dropped by half. Patients are getting a different type of dementia post-ART; this dementia is associated more with deficits in complex reasoning and less with global impairment. In addition, even though the incidence is dropping, HAD is occurring in patients with higher CD4 counts.

Myopathy in AIDS is uncommon and usually due to zidovudine (ZDV, AZT). Patients present with a generalized (proximal > distal) weakness and an elevated CPK.

Treatment is to stop the AZT.

Poliomyelitis is more likely to occur in AIDS patients. Differentiation between AZT myopathy and poliomyelitis may require muscle biopsy.

Peripheral AIDS neuropathy has 2 forms:

1) In chronic inflammatory demyelinating polyneuropathy, there is progressive weakness of the legs and loss of deep tendon reflexes. There is a high protein level and a high cell count in the patient's CSF. Treatments are corticosteroids, IVIG, and plasmapheresis—all equally effective.

2) Distal symmetric polyneuropathy is common in AIDS patients (1/3 get it). Symptoms are paresthesias of the feet and distal weakness in the legs. Treatment usually includes tricyclic antidepressants or gabapentin.

Progressive multifocal leukoencephalopathy (PML; affects white matter only) is usually seen in patients with T-cell immune defects (HIV/AIDS, chronic steroids, monoclonal antibodies). In addition, we are now seeing cases of PML in patients taking a number of immunosuppressants for treatment of rheumatologic, hematologic, and inflammatory bowel diseases (rituximab, fludarabine, mycophenolate, chronic corticosteroids), and with the newer drug to treat multiple sclerosis, natalizumab.

PML is caused by the human JC polyomavirus, resulting in a progressive demyelination of the CNS white matter.

Symptoms are varied and usually start with abnormal mentation and then slurred speech.

Diagnose with brain biopsy. Finding JC virus in the CSF by PCR is supportive (although this occurs less often in patients with PML who are being treated with ART).

Vacuolar myelopathy causes progressive weakness, incontinence, hyperreflexia, and ataxia. There is vacuolation and deterioration of the dorsal and lateral spinal columns. It is uncommon. This myelopathy must be differentiated from spinal cord compression due to some other cause, such as lymphoma.

PARASITIC CNS INFECTIONS

Toxoplasmosis

AIDS-related brain lesions: If you see multiple ring-enhancing lesions, think toxoplasmosis (CNS lymphoma, TB, or bacterial infections are less likely).

Because toxo is a reactivation infection, patients usually have IgG (but not IgM) antibody to *T. gondii*. But many people have toxo antibodies, so a positive toxo IgG is only supportive and not diagnostic. Also know that an absent toxo IgG does not exclude toxo as the cause of a brain lesion in an AIDS patient.

Treat with sulfadiazine, pyrimethamine, and leucovorin. Add dexamethasone if there's midline shift or rapid deterioration.

Do a brain biopsy if there is no improvement after empiric treatment, if there is a mass effect, or if there is only 1 lesion. Some empirically treat single lesions if the CD4 count is < 100 and the patient hasn't been on toxo prophylaxis. Relapses occur often.

Neurocysticercosis

Neurocysticercosis is the most common worldwide parasitic CNS infection. It is caused by ingesting food or water contaminated with *Taenia solium* (a tapeworm). It forms cysts in the brain, which initially cause no symptoms. But when the cyst walls break down several years later, it causes cerebral edema, usually with seizures as the first symptom.

MRI is the preferred imaging modality—when worms are viable, MRI shows multiple, non-enhancing hypodense lesions. As the worms die, they are surrounded by edema and flair. When dead, they calcify and shrink. Support the diagnosis with *T. solium* antibody testing on serum.

Treatment of CNS infection is controversial because of lack of randomized studies and propensity of dying worms to cause symptoms. Most experts now treat with high-dose praziquantel or albendazole +/– corticosteroids. AEDs are given to patients at high risk for seizures. More about this in the Infectious Disease section.

FUNGAL CNS INFECTIONS

Cryptococcal Meningitis

Especially consider cryptococcal meningitis when working up meningeal signs in AIDS patients and patients on chronic corticosteroids. CSF pressure is usually very elevated. Standard CSF studies can be entirely normal, so always check the cryptococcal antigen titer.

Treat with amphotericin B deoxycholate or liposomal ampho B and flucytosine x 2 weeks, then change to oral fluconazole x 8 more weeks (minimum). Lower doses of oral fluconazole are required for secondary prophylaxis in immunosuppressed patients. Manage elevated intracranial pressures with daily taps to keep CSF pressure < 200 mm H_2O, or patients can lose their vision. Shunts are appropriate if daily taps are needed. Do not use mannitol, acetazolamide, or corticosteroids. More about this in the Infectious Disease section.

STROKE

OVERVIEW

A stroke is defined as an infarcted area of the brain that results from any one of the following:

- Abnormal blood vessels (atherosclerosis)
- An embolism from the heart or extracranial vessels
- Reduced blood flow (hypotension or increased viscosity)
- Vessel rupture (hemorrhage)

Infarction results in cognitive, motor, and/or sensory deficits that can be temporary or permanent.

The same processes above (except for hemorrhage) can result in episodes of ischemia without infarction. Brain ischemia without infarction is a transient ischemic attack (TIA). The latest guidelines on TIA from the American Stroke Association (2009) have removed all references to duration of symptoms. The definition was changed because sometimes true infarction occurs even when symptoms last less than 24 hours, making the previous definition of TIA occasionally incorrect.

Strokes are classified as ischemic or hemorrhagic. Ischemic strokes can be thrombotic or embolic.

IMAGING OF STROKES

In 2009, the American Heart Association published recommendations for how best to image patients with possible stroke, based on an extensive literature review and specialty consensus publications. The recommendations focus on the best use of CT and MRI.

A main reason to do neuroimaging is to determine whether a patient is eligible for recombinant tissue plasminogen activator (rt-PA). Other uses:

- Image the cerebral parenchyma to:
  - Exclude intracerebral (ICH) or subarachnoid hemorrhage (SAH)
  - Detect ischemia
  - Exclude other illnesses that present as stroke
- Image the vessels
- Assess possible viability of infarcted tissue

Imaging with CT: a non-enhanced CT (NECT) scan can be performed as a basic form of stroke imaging (Image 11-4). The NECT can be enhanced by adding:

- Angiography (CTA) or
- Dynamic perfusion studies (CTP)

When adding angiography, evaluation of source images (SI) helps to interpret the study (CTA-SI).

Imaging with MRI: MRI can also be enhanced using additional imaging sequences:

- Diffusion weighted imaging (DWI)
- Perfusion (MRP)
- Angiography (MRA)
- Gradient-recalled echo (GRE)
- Fluid-attenuated inversion recovery (FLAIR)

The CT and MRI enhancements help to better accomplish the purposes of imaging. Usually most, if not all, of these sequences are performed whenever you order an MRI of the brain.

In the best circumstances, a CT scan with enhancements takes the same amount of time as an MRI

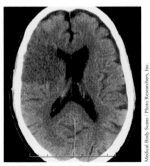

Image 11-4: CT of MCA stroke

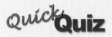

with enhancements. For example: It takes 10 minutes to do either NECT with CTA/CTA-SI and dynamic CTP or MRI with FLAIR, GRE, MRP, and intracranial MRA!

The major problem today is that not all hospitals provide access to the MRI scanner for triage situations. In many Emergency Departments, only CT is available.

Now that you know the acronyms, we'll go over which imaging to use in particular situations.

- Intracerebral hemorrhage (ICH): MRI-GRE is equivalent to NECT for finding blood. We used to believe that CT was better, but many studies now show that it is not. MRI is also better for detecting hemorrhagic transformation of ischemic stroke.
- Subarachnoid hemorrhage (SAH): Use NECT. MRI with FLAIR is probably as good as NECT, but as of now, we do not have any direct comparison studies.
- Ischemia: MRI-DWI is best. CTA-SI is comparable, but it is not as good for imaging of the posterior fossa/brain stem and for discovering small infarcts. MRI is also better than NECT to detect an occluded vessel.

Because of the above, unless your patient has signs and symptoms of SAH, MRI + DWI and GRE sequences (at minimum) is the best imaging for possible ischemic stroke because it both excludes ICH and identifies areas of infarction—provided you can get the test without delay. Remember that time from symptom onset > 4.5 hours precludes use of rt-PA (< 3 hours best). If you cannot get an MRI in a reasonable time frame, then get a CT with CTA-SI.

CTA or MRA is recommended to evaluate the intra- and extracranial vasculature of patients with TIA or stroke symptoms. Both imaging modalities are significantly more sensitive and specific than carotid Doppler ultrasound for diagnosing extracranial vascular stenosis. Carotid ultrasound also tends to overdiagnose lesions and leads to unnecessary surgery in some patients. CTA is better than MRI at identifying intracranial aneurysms.

If performing CTA or MRA doesn't extend the time period from symptom onset out past 4.5 hours maximum (< 3 hours best), either is recommended as part of the initial evaluation of stroke because, sometimes, clotted vessels can be treated with urgent intraarterial therapy or stents. Patients with a large clotted vessel—often the MCA, so-called "hard thrombus"—do not respond as well to rt-PA as direct intervention.

Although assessing viable brain tissue after infarction is one of the main purposes for imaging a stroke patient, we are still in the beginning stages of learning how to incorporate the data into treatment plans. Dynamic CTP and MRP are the leading imaging techniques.

ISCHEMIC STROKES

Thrombotic vs. Embolic Strokes

Thrombotic strokes: Atherosclerotic occlusion is most common in the internal carotid, middle cerebral, vertebral, and basilar arteries.

The initial neurologic symptoms often occur in a slow, stepwise progression (termed "stroke in evolution"). Often patients have a history of TIAs in the same distribution as the presenting symptoms of their stroke. If the patient has not had TIAs, a clear differentiation between thrombotic and embolic may be difficult. Other, rarer causes of thrombotic occlusion are lupus anticoagulant, polycythemia, meningovascular syphilis, dissecting aortic aneurysm, and thrombocytosis.

Embolic strokes: Neuro deficit is usually worst at onset. Embolic strokes are usually not preceded by a TIA. Emboli from the heart usually go to the middle > posterior > anterior cerebral arteries.

Anterior Circulation

Anterior Cerebral Artery (ACA) Strokes

When the ACA is affected, the weakness and sensory loss affect primarily the contralateral leg. Urinary incontinence and gait abnormalities may also be present. If the corpus callosum is affected, patients may have a tactile agnosia.

Buzzphrase: The patient with the ACA stroke typically presents with unilateral leg weakness.

Middle Cerebral Artery (MCA) Strokes

MCA strokes result in contralateral weakness (hemiplegia), sensory loss (hemianesthesia), and a homonymous hemianopsia. If the dominant hemisphere is involved (the left side in most people, even left-handed individuals), these patients experience aphasia.

A lesion that affects the lower part of the left frontal lobe (Broca's area) causes an expressive, or Broca's, aphasia. These patients understand language, but they have trouble forming words and sentences, so their speech is non-fluent and effortful. A lesion at the boundary of the temporal and parietal lobes causes a "fluent" aphasia, called Wernicke aphasia. These patients can't comprehend written or spoken language and have errors in their spontaneous speech (often speaking in "neologisms," which are invented words). If the non-dominant hemisphere is involved, they may experience changes in spatial perception and may develop hemineglect syndrome.

With parietal lesions of either hemisphere, "cortical" sensory signs (contralateral loss of two-point discrimination, sensory inattention, astereognosis, and agraphesthesia) are often present. Note: Sensory inattention means they don't perceive tactile stimuli contralateral to the involved hemisphere when stimuli are presented to both sides simultaneously. Astereognosis is a synonym for "tactile agnosia" and means they can't recognize objects by touching them. Agraphesthesia means they can't recognize numbers or letters when drawn on their palms.

If the lesion involves the frontal lobe, the patient may have a gaze preference or gaze deviation—they look toward the side of the lesion for 1–2 days after the stroke.

Buzz phrases: The patient with the MCA stroke typically presents with garbled speech and arm/leg weakness that is opposite the side of the stroke.

Posterior Circulation

Posterior Cerebral Artery (PCA) Stroke

PCA strokes usually cause contralateral homonymous hemianopsia (usually a superior quadrantanopsia with temporal lobe lesions, an inferior quadrantanopsia with parietal lobe lesions, or a homonymous hemianopsia with medial occipital lesions). There may be mild contralateral sensory loss, color anomia, and/or memory loss. If the patient has anomia for colors, the posterior aspect of the corpus callosum (splenium) may have been affected.

If disruption of blood flow occurs bilaterally, the memory loss is severe and persistent.

Bilateral cortical blindness may result from simultaneous or successive posterior cerebral artery occlusion but may also be due to anoxia related to surgery, especially cardiac surgery. Occasionally, patients with cortical blindness deny their visual defect (Anton syndrome).

Buzzphrase: The patient with PCA stroke typically presents with visual field defects + color blindness + paresthesias without any motor findings.

Single Hemisphere Strokes

Single hemisphere strokes usually do not affect paraspinal muscles or muscles of the pharynx, jaw, and forehead. If these muscles are affected, think bilateral hemispheric involvement or brainstem stroke (below).

Vertebral/Basilar Artery Occlusion

Vertebral and/or basilar artery occlusion is the usual cause of brainstem strokes. That the problem involves the posterior circulation delivering blood to brainstem (posterior fossa) structures is suggested by the following:

- Bilateral extremity motor and sensory dysfunction (quadriplegia in severe cases)
- "Crossed" motor and sensory findings (e.g., right face, left arm)
- Horner syndrome
- Cerebellar signs
- Stupor and coma
- Cranial nerve dysfunction not usually affected by single hemisphere strokes (diplopia, pharyngeal weakness, jaw weakness, and deafness)

A vertebral stroke may cause lateral medullary syndrome (also called Wallenberg syndrome), which has a mixed bag of symptoms [Know]:

- Ipsilateral cerebellar signs and symptoms (due to involvement of the inferior cerebellar peduncle and cerebellum)
- Nausea, vomiting, nystagmus (vestibular nuclei)
- Ipsilateral Horner syndrome (due to involvement of the descending sympathetic fibers)
- Ipsilateral palate and vocal cord weakness (involvement of the nucleus ambiguus)
- "Crossed" sensory loss (ipsilateral face and contralateral body, due to involvement of the trigeminal nucleus and tract and spinothalamic tract, respectively)

Buzzphrases: The patient with the posterior circulation stroke typically presents with:

- Dizziness and "seeing double" (if vertebrobasilar artery; sometimes with antecedent TIA symptoms)
- Lateral medullary syndrome (defined above)
- Vertigo + nystagmus + nausea + ataxia (if cerebellar)

(There are other brainstem infarction syndromes, but we won't discuss them here.)

Lacunar Infarcts

Small artery disease, usually due to chronic hypertension or diabetes, can lead to occlusion of very small arterioles with resultant small areas of brain necrosis. Over time, resorption of these necrotic regions causes small cysts or "lacunae" to develop.

Although most are silent, hallmarks of symptomatic lacunar infarcts are:

- Pure hemiplegia (with no sensory dysfunction)
- Pure hemisensory stroke (with no motor dysfunction)
- Ataxic hemiparesis (ataxia ipsilateral to hemiparesis)
- Clumsy hand-dysarthria syndrome

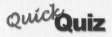

NEUROLOGY

- How does a patient with a PCA stroke typically present?

- What are the signs and symptoms of Wallenberg syndrome? What type of stroke causes it?

- When should you perform a lumbar puncture in a patient with possible stroke?

Multiple bilateral frontal lobe lacunae can result in pseudobulbar palsy: emotional incontinence with uninhibited crying or laughter, typically associated with a brisk jaw jerk.

Evaluation of Ischemic Stroke

The patient with a neurodeficit should be assessed like any other emergency, using the ABCs first: stabilize airway, breathing, and circulation. If the patient is stable, take a good history. The most important element is the time of symptom onset because that determines eligibility for an IV thrombolytic. If the patient awoke with deficits, then the last time she remembers having normal function is the time of symptom onset. Remember that complicated migraines, postictal states, and subdural hemorrhages can resemble a stroke, so ask about headaches, seizure activity, and falls.

Physical exam focuses on possible sources and alternative diagnoses. Look for evidence of seizures (tongue biting), trauma, myocardial ischemia, anterior and posterior carotid bruits, heart murmurs, and arrhythmias.

The National Institutes of Health Stroke Scale (NIHSS) score is a standardized instrument incorporated as part of a physical exam at most stroke centers. We've reproduced the general concepts of the scale in Table 11-3, but you really should study and use the full scale (which would take several pages to reproduce). A link to the NIHSS instrument is at the bottom of the table.

The NIHSS helps to quantify neurodeficits, communicate with neurologists, possibly identify the occluded vessel, make an early prognosis, and identify a patient's suitability for thrombolytics. Patients get points for their inability to complete the various parts of the assessment.

Recommended diagnostic tests at presentation of possible ischemic stroke include:

- Basic chemistries with glucose
- CBC with platelets
- PT, PTT, INR
- 12-lead ECG

Optional tests: A lumbar puncture with CSF assessment should be done if SAH is a concern and NECT does not show blood. Also consider an EEG (if you suspect patient has seizures), a urine drug screen, blood alcohol, blood gas, and pregnancy test as other potentially appropriate tests.

Treatment of Ischemic Stroke

If the stroke occurred < 3 hours ago and the NIH stroke scale is > 4, rt-PA has been shown to be effective in decreasing severity or reversing neurological deficits, provided that the patient fits a specific clinical presentation (2007 stroke treatment guidelines from the American Stroke Association).

Table 11-3: NIH Stroke Scale	
Assessment	**Instructions**
Consciousness: Level	Choose a response: Alert, arousable by minor stimuli, requires repeated or painful stimuli, unresponsive or reflexes only, or areflexic.
Consciousness: Questions	Ask month and age. No partial credit. Aphasic and stuporous patients score 2. Intubated patients score 1.
Consciousness: Commands	Ask patient to open and close eyes then to grip and release non-paretic hand.
Gaze	Test horizontal eye movements.
Vision	Test visual fields by confrontation with finger counting.
Facial palsy	Ask patient to show teeth or raise eyebrows and close eyes.
Motor: Arm and Leg	Test for pronator drift.
Ataxia	Perform finger-nose-finger and heel-shin tests.
Sensation	Assess for sensation or grimace to pinprick or withdrawal from noxious stimulus.
Language	Describe what is happening in a picture, name items printed on paper, and read a sentence.
Speech	Read words from a list.
Extinction and Inattention	Assess previous tests to determine if patient orients only to one side.
For the full scale with scoring, go to www.ninds.nih.gov/doctors/NIH_Stroke_Scale.pdf	

The following patients should be treated with rt-PA. The list also contains exclusion criteria for patients with stroke symptoms < 3 hours:

- Ischemic stroke with neurologic deficit(s) that is/are not minor or spontaneously improving
- No symptoms of subarachnoid hemorrhage or history of intracranial hemorrhage
- No head trauma, stroke, or myocardial infarct in last 90 days
- No GI or GU hemorrhage in last 21 days
- No major surgery in last 14 days
- No arterial punctures in last 7 days
- Systolic BP < 185 and diastolic BP < 110 mmHg
- No bleeding or trauma on exam
- Not taking oral anticoagulation, or INR ≤ 1.7 if taking anticoagulant
- Normal PTT if received heparin in past 48 hours
- Platelets ≥ 100,000/mm^3
- Blood glucose ≥ 50 mg/dL
- No history of seizures with postictal impairment
- CT area of infarct should be < 1/3 of middle cerebral artery territory
- Patient and/or family understand risks:benefits ratio

If > 3 hours but < 4.5 hours have elapsed, new data and recommendations from the American Stroke Association 2009 say patients can still be treated with rt-PA and receive benefit, provided that the following patients or situations are excluded (presence of any one excludes rt-PA):

- Age > 80 years
- Taking oral anticoagulants, regardless of INR
- Baseline National Institutes of Health Stroke Scale score > 25
- Comorbid diabetes mellitus

For stroke symptoms present for > 4–4.5 hours, management is conservative and emphasizes supportive care and treatment of complications:

- Give airway support to stroke patients with reduced consciousness or airway compromise; oxygen prn.
- Look for and treat sources of fever. Give antipyretics to reduce fever.
- Use cardiac monitoring for first 24 hours after stroke to assess for arrhythmias.
- Treat hypertension cautiously, so as not to extend infarct size. If the patient meets criteria for rt-PA except for BP, go ahead and give a drug to reduce BP to ≤ 185/110, then give rt-PA. If not giving rt-PA, withhold meds for BP < 220/120 and allow the patient to gradually drop their pressure on their own. If BP > 220/120, then treat with the goal of reducing the BP ~ 15% in first 24 hours. Recommended meds from guidelines include: IV labetalol, nitropaste, and nicardipine infusion.

- Restart antihypertensives for patients with long-standing hypertension after 24 hours (if not treated already for BP > 220/120).
- Maintain normoglycemia.

If the stroke occurs in the posterior fossa, admit the patient for close observation. Expansion of the contents of the posterior fossa can cause either upward or downward herniation, and these patients then decompensate quickly and without warning.

HEMORRHAGIC STROKE

Overview

Hemorrhagic stroke is usually due to bursting of small arteries, especially when the small artery branches off at a 90-degree angle from the parent vessel and the blood pressure is very high. The 2 most common causes are hypertension and amyloid angiopathy. Warfarin use is a risk factor, especially when the INR > 3.

Some patients have preexisting evidence of intermittent, small bleeds on MRI of the brain. It is possible that these MRI-visible "microbleeds" are indicators of which patients are prone to future intracerebral hemorrhage. Because the bleeding arises from small arteries, the symptoms usually evolve gradually but continuously.

Signs and Symptoms

Hemorrhagic stroke occurs in the following 4 areas of the brain (from most common site to least common):

1) **Putamen** and adjacent **internal capsule** (50%). If the hematoma involves the internal capsule, there is contralateral hemiparesis and usually sensory loss and hemianopsia. This type of hemorrhage may be difficult to distinguish from a middle cerebral artery infarct (one of the reasons to do the enhanced NECT or MRI looking for blood at presentation).
2) **Thalamus**: Contralateral hemianesthesia without "cortical" sensory signs. Some motor signs may be present if the adjacent internal capsule is involved.
3) **Pons**: Coma, pinpoint pupils, and quadriplegia. There may be decerebrate posturing bilaterally.
4) **Cerebellum**: Acute dizziness, ataxia, and vomiting with no change in mentation and no loss of consciousness.

Amyloid angiopathy is a common cause of hemorrhagic stroke after the 5th decade of life. The hemorrhage tends to be lobar and subcortical (Image 11-5). It rarely involves the deep structures (as does a hypertensive bleed). Hemorrhages may recur within months or years. Dementia occurs in 30%.

Remember: There are other causes of intracranial hemorrhage, including bleeding diatheses, trauma, and bleeding

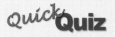

Quick Quiz

- Why should you keep a patient with an ischemic stroke to the posterior fossa under close observation?
- Where is the most common site for a cerebral hemorrhage?
- How does a pons stroke present?
- How does a cerebellar stroke present?
- Describe the typical symptoms of a subarachnoid hemorrhage.
- After an SAH, when is the patient most likely to rebleed?

into a tumor mass. Know that cocaine has been associated with development of vascular malformations and aneurysms that can be associated with major bleeding during episodes of severe drug-induced hypertension.

Treatment of Hemorrhagic Stroke

Treatment includes the basic supportive care given to ischemic stroke patients (see page 11-17).

Any anticoagulant effects should be immediately reversed with both vitamin K and replacement of clotting factors, no matter the reasons for anticoagulation. Give protamine for any hemorrhage associated with unfractionated heparin. Also stop any antiplatelet agents.

Control of intracranial pressure (ICP) is important, and mannitol is usually used.

Current guidelines to manage blood pressure recommend continuous IV antihypertensives (e.g., labetalol, nicardipine, enalapril) if SBP > 220 mmHg or MAP > 150 mmHg. For those with SBP 180–220 (MAP 130–150) and increased ICP, consider intermittent or continuous antihypertensives, keeping the perfusion pressure 31–80 mmHg.

Depending on the site of bleed, some clots should be surgically removed. Neurosurgeons are usually consulted.

SUBARACHNOID HEMORRHAGE

Overview

Subarachnoid hemorrhage (SAH) usually results from bleeding from an intracranial aneurysm. Aneurysms are most common at the bifurcation of vessels in the Circle of Willis or its major branches. The age when this most likely

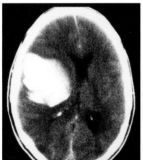

Image 11-5: CT of acute intra-cerebral hematoma

occurs is between 40 and 60, and it occurs in women more than men. The majority occur in the anterior circulation: 40% of aneurysms affect the internal carotid artery, 35% involve the anterior cerebral artery, and 20% the middle cerebral artery. Subarachnoid hemorrhage can also occur after a parenchymal bleed, when there is rupture into the ventricular system. Non-aneurysmal causes of SAH are rare but include AV malformations, sickle cell disease, bleeding diatheses, pituitary apoplexy, trauma, cocaine abuse, and intracranial arterial dissection.

The characteristic symptoms of SAH are the acute "thunderclap" or "worst headache of my life" sensation in combination with neck stiffness. Common associated symptoms include loss of consciousness, nausea/vomiting, and photophobia. More than 1/3 of patients report a history of "sentinel bleed" symptoms days or weeks earlier. The most important determinant of outcome is the neurological condition of the patient upon arrival at the hospital. If comatose, the prognosis is poor.

Diagnosis of SAH

NECT is the best test to identify blood in the subarachnoid space. If this is negative and the NECT does not show a mass, then do a lumbar puncture. The CT misses progressively more subarachnoid bleeds as time passes from initial rupture—picking up only about 50% of bleeds after 5 days. In a SAH, CSF is bloody with xanthochromic supernatant (pink or yellow tint); however, even clear CSF does not preclude the diagnosis because it may take hours after onset of the bleed before you find red cells in the CSF.

If a bleed is still suspected in the setting of a normal NECT and LP, then angiography is the procedure of choice. CTA and MRA are alternatives to invasive angiography, and their sensitivity/specificity is close to the standard angiogram. CTA is now very often included as an enhancement to the basic triage NECT for patients with stroke symptoms. The NECT in Image 11-6 shows a massive subarachnoid hemorrhage in which all the white in the brain tissue is due to blood in the subarachnoid space.

Complications of SAH

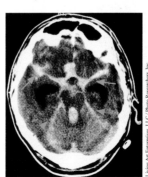

Image 11-6: Massive subarachnoid hemorrhage

After a sentinel bleed, rebleeding is common. The risk is highest in the first 24 hours, but the risk remains high for at least one month. Vasospasm may occur in up to 70% of patients and begins 3–5 days after the hemorrhage. It reaches a peak at 5–14 days and resolves in 2–4 weeks. The third major complication is communicating hydrocephalus, which occurs in 15–20% of patients after SAH. The likelihood of hydrocephalus depends on the volume of intraventricular and subarachnoid blood. Seizures occur in 5–10%; 2/3 begin within the 1st month after the hemorrhage, while the remaining occur within the 1st year.

Treatment of SAH

If the patient is on an anticoagulant or antiplatelet agent, stop the drug before performing any interventions. Surgical clipping or inserting a coil into the bleeding vessel are the major interventions used to prevent the aneurysm from bleeding again. Remaining treatment focuses on preventing the complications. Control of ICP and blood pressure is important as well, although recommendations are less clear-cut than with intracranial hemorrhages.

Other aneurysms: Mycotic aneurysms are caused by septic emboli, most often from infected heart valves. They are usually small and occur in the distal vasculature. This is in contrast to saccular aneurysms that occur more proximally, at the branch points of the arteries (at the point where the middle cerebral artery branches off of the internal carotid artery).

Know that first-degree relatives of patients who experienced a SAH have a 2–5x increased risk of a SAH. Consider aneurysmal screening in patients who have 2 or more relatives with SAH (or 1 relative with a diagnosis of autosomal dominant polycystic kidney disease). CTA or MRA are good, noninvasive tests.

SUBDURAL HEMATOMA

Subdural hematoma (SDH) is not always due to direct trauma, since deceleration forces can also cause it. But consider SDH in patients with a history of falls, blows to the head, and vehicle accidents. Subdural bleeds are usually of venous origin.

Half of the patients will immediately become comatose, but the other half will remain lucid for a time period of hours to days, after which cognition becomes gradually and progressively impaired until coma develops. Symptoms may also be fluctuating. Other signs of increased ICP are often present, such as headache, nausea/vomiting, neck stiffness, and gait abnormalities.

NECT is used in triage of these patients, but MRI with FLAIR is the most sensitive. NECT in Image 11-7 shows a subdural hematoma with a skull deformity.

Treatment for SDH is typically surgery.

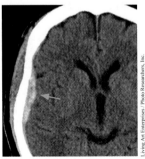

Image 11-7: Subdural hematoma

EPIDURAL HEMATOMA

Epidural hematomas, because of their arterial origin, evolve more rapidly than subdural hematomas. These are usually caused by temporal trauma that damages the middle meningeal artery—in association with temporal bone fractures. Symptoms of increased ICP are typically rapid after the head trauma, but a short period of lucidity may develop, followed by rapid obtundation.

As with SDH, diagnosis can be accomplished with NECT, but MRI with FLAIR is most sensitive.

Treatment consists of early evacuation of the hematoma via a craniotomy. If untreated, herniation occurs, with mortality varying from 15% to 40%.

TRANSIENT GLOBAL AMNESIA

Transient global amnesia (TGA) is characterized by abrupt onset of global anterograde amnesia, with a variable impairment of retrograde memory not associated with any other major neurologic signs or symptoms. Except for amnesia during and around the event, patients recover completely in 2/3 of cases within 2–12 hours and in almost all within 24 hours. It is considered benign, and the condition recurs infrequently.

Patients are usually between the ages of 50 and 80 years and suddenly develop an inability to make new memories, and, they act disoriented—asking multiple questions repeatedly. The amnesia can extend back to even years, although more commonly just days to weeks. Some patients have accompanying nausea and dizziness. TIA can present similarly and should be considered.

Precipitating events are seen in many cases and include strenuous exercise, intense emotion, sexual intercourse, pain, temperature extremes (swimming in cold water), cervical manipulation, coughing spells and other Valsalva-like activities, and medical procedures. The etiology is unknown, although migraine may predispose.

NECT and brain MRI with DWI are usually normal. PET and SPECT studies have shown hypoperfusion and hypometabolism in the hippocampi and associated mesial temporal lobe structures during the attack, with resolution following the attack. The attacks self-resolve. No treatment is necessary. Thiamine is often administered.

CNS METASTASES

CNS metastases typically cause a slow onset of symptoms (headaches, focal neuro deficits, impaired cognition, seizures, and/or stroke symptoms), although they can be abrupt if there is hemorrhage into a tumor.

Know the following (summarized in Table 11-4):

Parenchymal brain metastases occur most commonly with lung, renal, and breast cancer, as well as with melanoma and lymphoma.

Dural metastases occur with breast and prostate cancer.

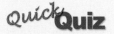

- Which evolve more quickly—eipidural or subdural hematomas? Why?
- A patient with history of prostate cancer and new onset of urinary incontinence should make you think of what type of problem?
- What is Wernicke encephalopathy? How is it treated?
- How does the presentation of the typical Wernicke patient differ from that of the typical Korsakoff patient?

Epidural metastases at the level of the spinal cord cause back pain, usually worse when lying down. New onset of bladder or bowel dysfunction (incontinence, urgency) is very important and should alert you to consider spinal epidural metastases, especially in the setting of new back pain. In a patient with a history of cancer, especially prostate, breast, and lung cancer, and cord compression symptoms, metastases must be ruled out!

Meningeal malignancy is most frequent in lymphomas, carcinoma of the breast, and melanoma. MRI with contrast is the best imaging study.

Treatment depends on how many metastases are present, the cancer prognosis, and the functional status of the patient. An approachable, single metastasis in a functional patient is treated with surgery and radiation. Small lesions (< 3 cm) and/or surgically inaccessible lesions can be treated with stereotactic radiosurgery. Less functional patients with numerous lesions are usually treated with whole brain radiation and chemotherapy +/– corticosteroids.

METABOLIC AND TOXIC DISORDERS

WERNICKE / KORSAKOFF

Wernicke encephalopathy and Korsakoff syndrome are considered different presentations of the same disease process. Wernicke's is milder and reversible while Korsakoff's is more severe and only partially reversible. The cause is thiamine (B_1) deficiency.

Wernicke encephalopathy is most often associated with alcoholism, but it can be seen in cases of malnutrition, malabsorption, increased requirements, and specific loss of thiamine during dialysis.

It is characterized by global confusion with inattention, apathy, disorientation, and memory loss that worsens over days to weeks. Abnormal eye movements are typical and include horizontal nystagmus and a disordered conjugate gaze that progresses to ophthalmoplegia (bilateral lateral rectus weakness, either in isolation or together with palsies of other extraocular muscles). The pupils may become sluggishly reactive to light. The person may have trouble standing or walking due to truncal ataxia. Diagnosis is clinical.

Know the typical Wernicke's presentation: confused + walks drunk + trouble moving eyes.

Korsakoff syndrome is often coincident with Wernicke's and may emerge as the symptoms of Wernicke's are treated. The amnesia that occurs with Korsakoff's can be both retrograde and anterograde. Attention and mentation appear normal. Patients will often confabulate because of the memory problems. The stories are frequently happy-go-lucky fantasies, so called "gleeful confabulation."

The typical Korsakoff's presentation: an underweight, poorly nourished but very attentive alcoholic who tells fantastical stories that couldn't possibly be true, then has no memory of the discussion.

Treatment. Immediate treatment with thiamine resolves the problem of Wernicke's and prevents Korsakoff syndrome. Once Korsakoff syndrome develops, thiamine has only partial effect. In fact, the majority of patients who emerge from Wernicke's have irreversible symptoms of Korsakoff's.

Treatment for Wernicke encephalopathy is thiamine, at a minimum dose of 500 mg (in saline) by infusion 3 times per day for 2–3 days, followed by 500 mg thiamine IV or IM daily for another 5 days. Thereafter, oral thiamine supplementation should be continued, typically at a dose of 100 mg/day. Deficiency in other vitamins and minerals, especially niacin and magnesium, should also be corrected. Wernicke's typically improves within hours of thiamine replacement.

In the Nephrology section, we discuss how IV glucose given to a chronic alcoholic causes a decrease in the already depleted stores of phosphate and can cause hypophosphatemia. A similar sequence can occur with the thiamine stores—IV glucose can precipitate Wernicke encephalopathy in alcoholics.

NEUROLOGY

Table 11-4: Main Mets to the Brain						
	Breast	**Lung**	**Prostate**	**Melanoma**	**Lymphoma**	**Renal**
Parenchymal	+	+		+	+	+
Dural	+		+			
Epidural	+	+	+			
Meningeal	+			+	+	

LITHIUM TOXICITY

Hyponatremia causes increased lithium resorption from the kidney. Toxic lithium levels cause seizures and coma; treat with hemodialysis.

ANTICHOLINERGIC TOXICITY

"Mad as a hatter." Dilated pupils, flushed, febrile, with secondary urinary retention.

See the General Internal Medicine section for more detail on these toxicities.

DISEASES OF MUSCLE AND NERVE

MYELOPATHIES

Myelopathies are diseases of the spinal cord. Typical manifestations are gait ataxia, spasticity, and hyper-reflexia. Bowel and bladder incontinence arise as disease worsens. There are many subcategories.

Metabolic Myelopathy

Subacute Combined Degeneration of Spinal Cord

Subacute combined degeneration of the spinal cord due to B_{12} deficiency is the prototype for metabolic myelopathy. Severe B_{12} deficiency causes segmental loss of myelin, especially in the dorsal and lateral columns. Clinical presentation is gradual weakness associated with paresthesias and loss of proprioception with development of ataxia. Severe cases end in extensive bilateral lower extremity weakness, spasticity, and urinary incontinence +/− cognitive impairment.

Cognitive changes include confusion, apathy, delusions, paranoia, and mental deterioration. Know that the neurologic changes can occur without any associated macrocytosis or anemia!

Diagnose by measuring serum B_{12}, methylmalonic acid (MMA), and homocysteine (HC) levels. MMA and HC are more sensitive tests that are included to make a diagnosis in patients who have low-normal or normal B_{12} levels. In states of B_{12} deficiency, both MMA and HC are increased.

Infectious Myelopathies

AIDS

Advanced AIDS patients can get a myelopathy with vacuolation and deterioration of the dorsal and lateral spinal columns that presents as ascending paresis with a sensory component (loss of vibration and proprioception) and urinary incontinence. Many other things can do this in a patient with virtually no immune system, but be sure to exclude a cord lesion with MRI.

Epidural Abscess

Spinal epidural abscess is a medical emergency that requires rapid diagnosis and treatment of the bacterial infection. The abscess can develop from bacteremic seeding from any source or contiguous infection after spine surgery. Risk factors include immunodeficiency states (e.g., diabetes, HIV/AIDS), alcoholism, and any conditions or behaviors associated with transient bacteremia (e.g., injection drug use and boils). The abscess may start as a spinal osteomyelitis and progress to an abscess, causing cord compression. *S. aureus* is the most common etiology of epidural abscess.

Remember: The main symptom of epidural abscess is back pain. Suspect epidural abscess in anyone who has been bacteremic from any cause and presents with back pain and fever. For example: Rule out epidural abscess in the postpartum patient who had an epidural during delivery—the cause is almost always some type of nosocomial *Staphylococcus* species.

Initial symptoms include a few days to 2 weeks of fever and backache with localized tenderness, radicular pain, and neurologic deficits. Not all patients have all of the symptoms.

Abscess is best diagnosed with immediate contrasted MRI with FLAIR (contrasted CT is a less-sensitive alternative), TB skin test, and blood cultures. Perform myelography if the abscess is not clearly seen by MRI (or CT, if that was the only option).

Treatment: Immediate decompression with laminectomy and drainage followed by appropriate antibiotics, except in cases of TB where treatment is entirely medical (using 4-drug antituberculous antimicrobials).

Tuberculosis

Pott disease is tuberculous osteomyelitis of the spine and is sometimes associated with cord compression. Usually, this form of TB is due to reactivation disease (rarely is it primary tuberculosis).

Clinical presentation is back pain, fever, weight loss, and possible neurologic deficits and/or radicular symptoms.

Diagnosis is made with a high index of suspicion, biopsies for pathology and culture, and a TB skin test.

Treatment is with standard 4-drug TB therapy (see the Pulmonary section for specific details).

Syphilis

Both secondary and tertiary syphilis can affect the cord. The secondary manifestation of meningovascular syphilis can present as stroke or as infarction of the spinal cord (rare). Tertiary syphilis presents as cognitive impairment, tabes dorsalis, and/or aortitis.

The cognitive impairment can be remembered by the mnemonic PARESIS: personality, affect, reflexes, eyes [Argyll-Robertson pupil], sensorium, intellect, speech.

Quick Quiz

- Describe the findings in subacute combined degeneration due to B_{12} deficiency.
- What bacteria is usually the cause of an epidural abscess?
- What is the best test to diagnose epidural abscess?
- What are the symptoms of cervical myelopathy?
- Lumbosacral myelopathy affects which dermatomes? Which myotomes? What are the findings on physical exam?
- What is lumbar spinal stenosis? What are the classic exacerbating and relieving body positions and movements?

Tabes dorsalis is syphilitic involvement of the posterior columns that causes deficits in proprioception, manifesting as ataxia and paresthesias.

Tabes dorsalis is diagnosed using the following:

- Screening tests for syphilis (RPR or VDRL)
- *T. pallidum*-specific testing (MHA-TP)
- +/– lumbar puncture and biopsies with routine path and cultures (more about syphilis in the Infectious Disease section)

Inflammatory Myelopathy

Transverse Myelitis (TM)

TM is inflammation of 1 or 2 segments of the cord (usually thoracic) as a post-infectious complication or from unknown causes. It is also associated with multiple sclerosis and several autoimmune disorders (lupus, mixed connective tissue disease, Sjögren's, scleroderma, rheumatoid arthritis).

Clinical presentation is most often acute, progressive, bilateral leg weakness with a sensory deficit below the level of the lesion, and paresthesias.

Contrasted MRI shows the inflammation. CSF analysis shows increased protein, lymphocytosis, and normal glucose. Treatment depends on the underlying cause (e.g., autoimmune disease vs. post-viral complication), but most patients recover some function after about 3 months. Steroids are controversial in idiopathic cases.

Compression-Induced Myelopathies

Cervical Spondylosis with Myelopathy

Cervical spondylosis (spinal osteoarthritis) with myelopathy begins with changes in the intervertebral discs. These changes occur gradually and accumulate with age. Neck pain is common. If the disc herniates, it will compress a nerve root, causing a radiculopathy at that level. Note: Radiculopathy is numbness, paresthesias, weakness, and hyporeflexia in the corresponding region that is supplied by the compressed nerve root.

When the spondylosis becomes more severe, it may compress the spinal cord itself, causing spasticity, hyperreflexia, and gait abnormalities.

If a rheumatoid arthritis patient presents with a post-op focal neuro deficit, suspect C1–2 spinal cord trauma induced by intubation. This is likely if the patient has chronic asymptomatic C1–2 subluxation. Anesthesiologists are generally well aware of this susceptibility. Of course, other mechanisms can cause similar injury in these patients.

Thoracic Myelopathy

Thoracic sensory levels: T4 at nipple line and T10 at umbilicus. Thoracic spondylosis is distinctly unusual. In thoracic myelopathies, think tumor or transverse myelitis, not compression.

Lumbosacral Myelopathy

Lumbosacral (LS): The cord ends at L1–2. Lumbosacral disease affects the cauda equina and nerve roots, usually causing L4, L5, or S1 radiculopathy.

Affected dermatomes:

- L5 = great toe (L5 = Large toe)
- S1 = lateral side of foot by the small toe (S1 = Side of foot near Small toe)

Affected myotomes:

- L5 = weakness of the great toe extensor and ankle dorsiflexion (patients have trouble standing on the heel and present with foot drop)
- S1 = weakness of ankle plantar flexion (patients have trouble standing on the toes)

Lumbar spinal stenosis is a congenital narrowing of the spinal canal in the area of T10–L1, the conus medullaris. Patients are more susceptible to impingement of the cauda equina secondary to disc disease, ligamentous degeneration, and arthritis.

Lumbar spinal stenosis may result in neurogenic claudication, characterized by a deep, progressive ache in the legs, sometimes associated with lower extremity numbness, paresthesias, or weakness, which is precipitated by standing or walking for a few minutes. These symptoms are aggravated by upright posture, which extends the spine, and are relieved by sitting or squatting (flexing hips/spine).

Buzz phrases that help you diagnose spinal stenosis include: "Gets better when bending over the shopping cart" or "improves when walking uphill." These activities curve the vertebral bodies and open space in the canal.

Differential diagnosis for spinal stenosis includes vascular claudication, which also causes symptoms when walking or exercising leg muscles but not when standing upright (Table 11-5).

Table 11-5: Spinal Stenosis vs. Claudication

	Change In Symptoms:		
	Walking	Standing	Sitting
Lumbar Spinal Stenosis	Worse	Worse	Better
Claudication	Worse	Better	Better

Confirm the diagnosis of lumbar spinal stenosis with an MRI. Treatment is conservative (physical therapy and analgesics). Surgery is a last resort for patients who have debilitating pain not relieved with conservative measures. Surgery is indicated urgently, however, in patients with progressive neurologic deficits or incontinence.

Miscellaneous Myelopathies

Syringomyelia

Syringomyelia is a progressive myelopathy caused by cavitation of the central spinal cord, typically in the cervical and thoracic regions. It can be idiopathic, developmental, or acquired. About 2/3 of cases are associated with Arnold-Chiari malformation—a congenital malformation in which there is a downward shift of the cerebellar tonsils and medulla through the foramen magnum into the cervical area of the spine, sometimes with syrinx (cyst) formation.

Symptoms of syringomyelia typically occur as a "suspended" or "cape-like" sensory deficit across the shoulders and proximal upper limbs. The patient initially has a relatively normal sense of light touch and vibration, but no sense of pain or temperature in the involved dermatomes, reflecting involvement of the crossing spinothalamic fibers in the central part of the cord. When the anterior horn is affected, weakness and atrophy of the upper limbs occur, starting in the hands and moving proximally to include the arms and then shoulder muscles. Occipital and nuchal headaches are also very common.

Diagnose syringomyelia with MRI.

Anterior Horn Cell Disorders

Anterior horn cell problems cause motor deficits only. Amyotrophic lateral sclerosis (ALS), or Lou Gehrig disease, is the most common cause of anterior horn cell disease. The hallmark of ALS is marked, simultaneous upper and lower motor neuron signs.

A patient with ALS has:

• Diffuse hyperreflexia and spasticity (upper motor neuron), along with
• Fasciculations, weakness, and atrophy (lower motor neuron)

Think about ALS in the patient who presents with weakness in the lower extremities (possibly even falls) and difficulty with fine motor skills, and who has fasciculations and/or atrophy on exam. Cognitive dysfunction is not a feature.

The disorder is relentlessly progressive, involving upper and lower extremities, truncal and bulbar musculature, and is terminal usually within 3–5 years after diagnosis. Management of these patients includes determining how to proceed with respiratory and nutritional support as the disease progresses.

Polio used to be the most common cause of anterior horn cell disease; now post-polio syndrome must also be considered. Post-polio syndrome causes areflexia and progressive weakness. "Spinal muscular atrophy" is a set of hereditary disorders of the anterior horn lower motor neurons. A polio-like presentation today is more likely to be due to West Nile virus encephalitis.

NEUROPATHIES

Overview

Neuropathies can be divided into several categories based on which nerves are affected.

If the process involves only 1 nerve, it is called mononeuropathy. Mononeuropathies are generally due to entrapment (as with carpal tunnel syndrome).

If 2 or more nerves are affected in a limited distribution, the term mononeuritis multiplex is used. Mononeuritis multiplex results from systemic disorders like diabetes or vasculitis.

Neuropathies that symmetrically and diffusely involve the peripheral nerves are called peripheral neuropathies (or polyneuropathy). There are many causes of peripheral neuropathy (see below).

The workup for any neuropathy includes glucose, ESR, creatinine, free T_4 and TSH levels, CBC, and a chest x-ray. Electromyography and nerve conduction studies (EMG/NCS) are done as a first step, regardless of whether the symptoms are mono- or polyneuropathy. EMG/NCS help to identify any disease of muscle and characterize nerve conduction. Serum protein electrophoresis, immunoglobulin electrophoresis, and quantitative immunoglobulin assays are also done if the patient is > 40 years old, particularly if the EMG/NCS suggest a demyelinating neuropathy.

Inflammatory and hereditary neuropathies are the most frequently missed causes of polyneuropathy. So consider inflammatory causes and include a careful family history in your evaluation of peripheral neuropathies!

Mononeuropathies

Focal / Compressive

Focal mononeuropathies are caused by localized peripheral nerve damage, usually from a compression injury (although ischemia can do it also, especially in autoimmune diseases associated with vasculitis). The main sites of compression are the ulnar nerve at the elbow, the median nerve at the wrist, and the peroneal nerve at the knee (discussed below). Because radiculopathies

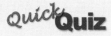

- From the patient's history, what clues help you differentiate lumbar spinal stenosis from vascular claudication?
- What part of the spinal cord does syringomyelia affect?
- What disease presents with both upper motor neuron and lower motor neuron deficits? How do people with this disease present?
- Where are the main points of compression for the ulnar, median, and peroneal nerves?
- Nocturnal awakening with hand pain is frequently due to what? What nerve does it affect? Where does the numbness occur?
- Is the ankle jerk normal or decreased with S1 radiculopathy? With sciatica?

and mononeuritis multiplex can have presentations similar or identical to focal compressive neuropathies, they must also be considered in the workup of patients presenting with focal neuropathic symptoms.

Acute **wrist drop** (radial neuropathy) is usually from nerve compression but is occasionally seen as a result of diabetic neuropathy (discussed below) and may also occur with lead toxicity. It has been called "Saturday night palsy" in inebriated patients because it occurs after bouts of unconsciousness whereby the nerve becomes compressed in the radial groove of the humerus. This usually resolves slowly over several weeks or months (provided the patient doesn't continually reinjure the nerve!). Physical therapy is the best treatment, using wrist splints.

Lower brachial plexus injury (2° surgery/tumor) causes a claw-hand deformity, similar to that which may be seen with severe ulnar neuropathy.

Carpal tunnel syndrome (CTS) is median nerve entrapment at the wrist, usually from repetitive stress, causing sensory loss, paresthesias, and weakness involving the first 3 or 4 digits of the hand, but patients can have pain anywhere in the arm or shoulder! Thenar muscle atrophy may occur. Median nerve entrapment at the wrist almost invariably causes nocturnal awakening due to hand pain or paresthesias (Image 11-8). Prevalence of hypothyroidism is 1–10% in patients with CTS, so most experts recommend screening with TSH.

Initial treatment of carpal tunnel syndrome is neutral alignment wrist splints and modifying the repetitive stress. If this is ineffective, steroid injection may help. Next step is median nerve release. Certain exercises (yoga and some specific physical therapy exercises such as "nerve gliding") seem to help. Ultrasound helps some.

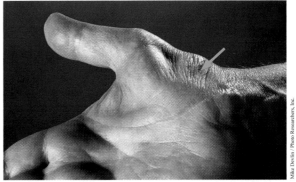

Image 11-8: Thumb muscle wasting due to carpal tunnel syndrome

Know that pregnancy can cause an acute presentation of CTS that typically improves after delivery. Splints are the best treatment for this patient group.

Ulnar neuropathy causes sensory loss and paresthesias in the little finger and ulnar aspect of the ring finger, as well as weakness of finger abductors and adductors. It is usually due to lesions at the elbow but also occurs at the entrance of the ulnar nerve to the cubital tunnel and at the wrist. Rarely, trauma to the heel of the hand can result in an ulnar injury. Elbow pads and splints help. Surgery is also an option for refractory cases.

Sciatic nerve compression causes pain and paresthesias that travel down the back or side of the leg into the foot or ankle. It can, like S1 radiculopathy, cause difficulty standing on toes. Unlike S1 radiculopathy, it does not cause a decreased ankle jerk when compared to the opposite ankle (Table 11-6).

Table 11-6: S1 Radiculopathy vs. Sciatica		
	Able to Tiptoe?	**Decreased Ankle Jerk?**
S1 Radiculopathy	No	Yes
Sciatica	No	No

Peroneal nerve compression. Compression usually occurs at the proximal head of the fibula, causing foot drop. Remember that L5 radiculopathy also causes foot drop.

To distinguish between peroneal nerve compression and L5 radiculopathy: Patients with peroneal nerve compression cannot evert the foot well but can still invert it, while L5 radiculopathy prevents or hinders both eversion and inversion (Table 11-7). Also, it is useful to test proximal L5 innervated muscles such as the hamstrings and thigh abductors, which will not be affected with peroneal nerve compression.

Know that Charcot-Marie-Tooth disease (see below) can cause symptoms similar to peroneal nerve compression.

Table 11-7: Radiculopathy vs. Peroneal Nerve Injury

	Foot Drop?	Able to Invert Foot?	Able to Evert Foot?
L5 Radiculopathy	Yes	No	No
Peroneal Nerve Injury	Yes	Yes	No

Mononeuritis Multiplex

Note that mononeuritis multiplex can present identically to the compressive focal neuropathies above. Rather than being caused by nerve compression, mononeuritis multiplex is caused by a systemic disease.

Consider any of the following as a possible cause of mononeuropathy +/– multiplex:

• Rheumatoid arthritis.
• DM.
• Connective tissue diseases.
• Vasculitis.
• Polyarteritis.
• Lyme disease (think of this in a hiker with new-onset foot drop). CNS Lyme disease is discussed in the Infectious Disease section.
• Neuralgic amyotrophy (see next).

Neuralgic amyotrophy (other names: Parsonage-Turner syndrome, brachial plexus neuropathy, acute brachial radiculitis) is temporary inflammation of the brachial plexus that may follow a vaccination or viral illness. Initially, it causes extreme pain in the shoulder with radiation to the arm, neck, and back. Within hours to days after the onset of pain, the shoulder muscles and proximal arm musculature become weak. Bilateral involvement may occur. Diagnosis is clinical, supported by EMG/NCS. It improves in 1–3 years with conservative management.

Bell Palsy

Bell palsy is caused by dysfunction of the external 7th cranial nerve. It is regarded as idiopathic, but herpes simplex (or its associated immune response) is the cause of most cases (definitively supported by finding evidence of the virus by PCR in the affected nerve roots).

Varicella zoster is also a cause and is the probable diagnosis when a clinical scenario includes vesicles involving the tympanic membrane and external auditory canal (Ramsay Hunt syndrome).

Two important systemic diseases can also cause a facial palsy that presents identically:

1) Lyme disease
2) Acute HIV

Some experts call these palsies "Bell's," but others prefer to identify them as a systemic manifestation of Lyme or HIV.

Bell palsy affects 1 side of the face, including the forehead. It causes ipsilateral facial muscle paralysis and occasionally results in no taste sensation on the anterior 2/3 of tongue, loss of lacrimation, and hyperacusis. Pregeniculate lesions are associated with the loss of taste, salivation, and lacrimation, while more distal lesions spare these functions.

To help differentiate Bell palsy from other nerve damage, know that cortical lesions spare the muscles of the forehead and upper eyelid, whereas Bell palsy affects them.

Diagnosis is clinical. Imaging of the head is reserved for patients who don't improve within 6 months or who continue to progress with facial weakness after 3 weeks. Know that if the palsy is preceded by a period of facial twitching, the risk of tumor is higher. These patients should have urgent imaging.

Patients who begin to improve within 3 weeks will usually recover completely. If complete ipsilateral paralysis occurs, full recovery is less likely.

A week of prednisone shortens the course and improves function if started within 7 days of clinical onset. Studies assessing combined antiviral drugs (acyclovir or valacyclovir) + prednisone show conflicting results. Some experts give both; others do not unless obvious signs of herpes are present; i.e., vesicles. Eyelid surgery is reserved for patients with severe palsy, or where there is corneal anesthesia or xerophthalmia not amenable to eye lubricants.

Diabetic Mononeuropathies

Know that diabetes is associated with several cranial neuropathies (III, VI, IV: present with eye pain, drooping eyelids, double vision; and VII-Bell's). Radial, ulnar, and peroneal isolated neuropathies are also more common in diabetics.

Note that diabetic involvement of the 3rd cranial nerve typically presents with double vision and weak eye movements without any changes in the pupils. Exam questions might have the patient presenting with diplopia and (pick one) chronic sensory dysfunction, wrist drop, or foot drop.

Polyneuropathies

Demyelinating vs. Axonal Polyneuropathies

Demyelinating polyneuropathies affect motor fibers and present primarily as weakness.

Axonal polyneuropathies are usually a sensorimotor combination, with sensory abnormalities appearing first (paresthesias progressing to numbness), then motor weakness appearing later.

Quick Quiz

- Can a patient with L5 radiculopathy evert the foot?
- What infection should you consider in a hiker from Connecticut who presents with new onset of foot drop?
- What CSF findings are typically seen in patients with Guillain-Barré syndrome?
- How does the treatment of CIDP differ from the treatment of Guillain-Barré syndrome?

Guillain-Barré Syndrome

Guillain-Barré Syndrome (GBS) is the most common autoimmune, inflammatory polyneuropathy. We now understand that GBS is a syndrome that contains demyelinating (most common) and axonal variants.

Classic demyelinating GBS (termed Acute Inflammatory Demyelinating Polyradiculoneuropathy, AIDP, 90% of U.S. cases) presents as an ascending paralysis, including pulmonary muscles, with areflexia. In practice, patients may have some mild sensory abnormalities and paresthesias, but usually on the exam questions, GBS is a pure motor illness with absent reflexes.

The Miller Fisher axonal variant (MFV, 5% of cases) is a type of GBS that includes only areflexia, ataxia, and ophthalmoplegia; e.g., patients present unable to move their eyes or walk upright.

Two other rare axonal variants comprise the remaining 5% of cases.

Know that the CSF has a normal cell count and a high protein—suspect another diagnosis if the CSF has more than 10 WBC/mm^3. EMG/NCS help to characterize the variant (axonal or demyelinating).

Anti-GQ1b IgG is a unique serum protein measurable in over 80% of MFV cases of GBS and assists with diagnosis of this variant.

The axonal variants are commonly associated with preceding Campylobacter jejuni infections and also development of many antibodies against the gangliosides found in peripheral nerves (anti-GM1, -GD1a, -GalNAC, -GD1a, -GD1b). These antibodies aren't routinely measured, however, except for anti-GQ1b.

Plasmapheresis and IV immunoglobulin therapy (IVIG) are equally effective. Use one or the other if patients present within 4 weeks of initial symptoms.

Do not use steroids because they do not work. Complete recovery is the norm for about 80%, but 20% of patients either progress and die on the ventilator (of other causes) or have significant residual weakness.

Chronic Inflammatory Demyelinating Polyneuropathy (CIDP)

The initial presentation of CIDP is similar to the AIDP variant of Guillain-Barré, but the disorder then follows a chronic relapsing or chronic progressive course and has a more significant sensory component. CIDP cases are usually not traceable to an inciting event, either. (Still, it's useful to think of CIDP as "Guillain-Barré that won't go away.") Consider CIDP in the patient with a demyelinating polyneuropathy (by EMG/NCS) that extends beyond 8 weeks in duration.

LP and EMG are identical to GBS (high protein, no pleocytosis, and demyelinating polyneuropathy). Exclude systemic disorders, specifically HIV, hepatitis viruses, Lyme, thyroid disease, diabetes, myeloma, sarcoid, and connective tissue disorders such as lupus.

Unlike in Guillain-Barré, glucocorticoids hasten recovery and prevent relapse in CIDP. Plasmapheresis or IVIG are also standard treatments (pick 1 of the 3). Several other immunomodulators have been used chronically.

Charcot-Marie-Tooth (CMT)

CMT is called hereditary motor and sensory neuropathy and is by far (90%) the most common inherited peripheral polyneuropathy. There are 7 "types" composed of > 30 separate disorders under the general heading of CMT, all caused by mutations in myelin genes that are inherited variably (autosomal dominant, autosomal recessive, or X-linked).

Know that CMT diseases are demyelinating and are differentiated based on genetic markers. All have both motor and sensory impairment and usually present within the first 2 decades of life. The really rare ones tend to cluster in families. Diagnosis is very simple with genetic testing, and most patients never even have to have EMG/NCS testing. Treatment is supportive.

Diabetic Peripheral Neuropathy (DPN)

DPN is an axonal neuropathy that mainly causes sensory changes, including pain. Over time (usually 1 year), however, the pain usually relents in favor of numbness.

Effective treatments for pain include the FDA-approved DPN drugs duloxetine (Cymbalta®) and pregabalin (Lyrica®)—both are equally effective. Other drugs that are used include tricyclic antidepressants, carbamazepine, gabapentin, lamotrigine, tramadol, and venlafaxine. Topical treatment with capsaicin cream and lidocaine also help.

Alcoholic Peripheral Neuropathy

Alcohol is directly toxic to both nerves and muscles and causes many kinds of neuropathies (peripheral, autonomic, compressive). The polyneuropathy is typically axonal but is made worse if demyelination is superimposed (caused by nutritional deficiencies).

Symptoms of alcoholic axonal neuropathy start with pain and numbness in the feet in a stocking distribution. Over time, patients lose reflexes, proprioception, and strength.

Patients slowly recover with multivitamin therapy and abstinence from alcohol.

Remember that acute thiamine deficiency presents as Wernicke's, a polyneuropathy (weakness of extraocular muscles and ataxia) associated with delirium.

Other Axonal Neuropathies

Other somewhat common (and Board-relevant) causes of axonal polyneuropathy:

- Toxins, such as heavy metals (lead, arsenic)
- Chemotherapy drugs (vincristine)
- Isoniazid
- B_6 (pyridoxine) overdose from nutritional supplements
- Organophosphates
- Systemic illnesses (myeloma, porphyrias, thyroid disease, hepatitis viruses, amyloidosis, and HIV/AIDS)

Time of Onset

Differentiating among the polyneuropathies is aided by the time of onset:

- **Short** time of onset (days) suggests porphyric, Guillain-Barré, and certain toxic polyneuropathies.
- **Long** onset (over several years) is seen with the hereditary disorders, such as Charcot-Marie-Tooth or CIDP.
- **Subacute** onset (several weeks to 2 years) occurs in the majority:
  ◦ Toxicity (lead and glue-sniffing cause mainly motor effects, while INH and vincristine cause sensorimotor effects)
  ◦ Nutritional deficiencies (especially B_1, B_6, and B_{12})
  ◦ Paraneoplastic (see Lambert-Eaton below)
  ◦ Rheumatologic disorders

NEUROMUSCULAR JUNCTION

MYASTHENIA GRAVIS (MG)

MG is an autoimmune disorder. Most patients have auto-antibodies to either the postsynaptic acetylcholine receptor or muscle-specific tyrosine kinase receptor (MuSK)! An even smaller group of MG patients has neither anti-acetylcholine receptor nor anti-MuSK antibodies (termed "seronegative MG"). Either or neither, but not both.

MG is associated with thymomas (~ 15% of patients) and thymic hyperplasia (~ 60%), although we do not understand exactly how the thymus is related to anti-body formation.

The 2 forms of MG are:

1) **Generalized MG**: The clinical presentation of generalized MG is episodic weakness with repetitive movements (weakness; not tiredness, not soreness).

Symptoms are worse at the end of the day. Common presenting complaints include weakness while brushing hair, putting away dishes or climbing stairs, and diplopia after a long day. Weakening with repetitive muscle stimulation during the physical exam suggests the diagnosis. Ptosis is common.

2) **Ocular MG** presents as weakness localized to the eyes (lids and extraocular muscles).

Diagnosis of myasthenia gravis is best confirmed by measuring acetylcholine receptor or MuSK antibodies. Patients with generalized myasthenia usually have 1 of the 2 antibodies, whereas 50% of patients with ocular myasthenia are seronegative. More often, anti-MuSK is present in patients who are negative for anti-acetylcholine receptor antibodies. Antibody levels are not necessarily prognostic, but they do rise and fall with immunotherapy.

The edrophonium (Tensilon®) test is available (after a brief shortage in 2008) but is usually not performed because results are not as reliable as antibody measurements.

Routine electrodiagnostic studies, including repetitive nerve stimulation studies and single-fiber EMG, are useful in supporting the diagnosis.

Do thyroid function studies because 30% of patients with myasthenia gravis have thyroid disease. Look out for symptoms that suggest lupus or rheumatoid arthritis, since there is considerable overlap. Image the chest with CT or MRI in all confirmed diagnoses to rule out thymoma.

Treatments used for myasthenia gravis:

- Anticholinesterase agents (pyridostigmine [Mestinon®])
- Immunomodulators in patients uncontrolled on pyridostigmine (steroids and others)
- IVIG or plasmapheresis (for myasthenic crisis only because duration of action is very short)
- Thymectomy (takes years to see effects but definitely perform in patients with thymoma)

Myasthenic crisis is, by definition, respiratory failure.

Know the few drugs that can precipitate myasthenic crisis in patients with either known or undiagnosed MG:

- Aminoglycosides
- Magnesium sulfate
- β-blockers
- Penicillamine
- Procainamide
- Quinidine
- α interferon

LAMBERT-EATON SYNDROME

Lambert-Eaton myasthenic syndrome is caused by small cell lung cancer (2/3) and autoimmune diseases. It is itself an autoimmune disease in which antibodies are produced that are specific for calcium channels in pre-synaptic peripheral nerve terminals—causing decreased release of acetylcholine from the nerve terminals.

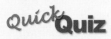

- Do the hereditary polyneuropathies have a short or long onset?
- How is myasthenia gravis diagnosed?
- What hormone tests do you always do for a patient with MG?
- What type of lung cancer causes Lambert-Eaton syndrome?
- What are the symptoms of Lambert-Eaton syndrome?
- What type of inflammatory myopathy does not respond to glucocorticoids?
- Where is the muscle weakness that occurs with inclusion body myositis?

Know the following about symptoms:

- Typical symptoms are gradually progressive proximal muscle weakness, aching thighs, dry mouth (autonomic dysfunction), and hyporeflexia, especially in the lower extremities.
- Lambert-Eaton syndrome rarely involves the ocular muscles.
- It looks like myasthenia gravis, except repetitive exercise may improve the weakness.

Diagnose Lambert-Eaton by measuring voltage-gated calcium-channel antibodies (anti-VGCC). Anti-VGCC antibodies are not 100% specific (they are sometimes found in patients who do not have Lambert-Eaton), so measure them only in patients who have a high pre-test probability of true disease. EMG can help distinguish between Lambert-Eaton and myasthenia (with decremental response to rapid stimulation in myasthenia and incremental response to rapid stimulation in Lambert-Eaton syndrome).

Look for malignancy in anybody diagnosed with Lambert-Eaton—especially small cell lung cancer.

Treatment includes treating any underlying malignancy along with drugs that increase the amount of acetylcholine in the synapse (guanidine, 3,4-diaminopyridine, and pyridostigmine). Refractory cases can be treated with IVIG or prednisone.

MYOPATHIES

Inflammatory myopathies:

- Dermatomyositis
- Polymyositis
- Inclusion body myositis

Both dermatomyositis and polymyositis usually cause:

- Elevated CPK
- Proximal muscle weakness

Both respond to corticosteroids.

Inclusion body myositis is a less common type of myositis in which patients present with:

- Elevated CPK
- Distal weakness (often hand)

It does not respond to corticosteroids. Muscle biopsy in inclusion body myositis shows vacuolar inclusions. More in the Rheumatology section on dermato-/polymyositis.

Endocrine myopathies: Proximal muscle weakness of varying degrees may be seen in patients with hyperthyroidism, hypothyroidism, parathyroid dysfunction, and adrenal and pituitary dysfunction. CPK is normal. Muscle biopsy usually shows Type 2 fiber atrophy, a nonspecific change.

Metabolic myopathies: A metabolic cause of muscle dysfunction is suggested by muscle fatigue, pain, cramping, and (in more severe cases) contractures and myoglobinuria, typically precipitated by exercise. The major categories are:

- Disorders of carbohydrate metabolism.
- Disorders of lipid metabolism.
- Disorders of mitochondrial function. Mitochondrial myopathies are distinguished by the presence of ragged red fibers on light microscopy of a muscle biopsy.

Duchenne muscular dystrophy is an X-linked disorder that causes progressive muscle weakness, starting at about 2 years of age and progressing to death as a young adult. The weakness is more proximal than distal. Look for an elevated CPK.

Myotonic dystrophy is the name of 2 types of inherited, adult-onset, neuromuscular disorders that have multisystem effects. The genetic abnormalities result in weakened skeletal muscle, cardiac conduction defects, cataracts, hypogonadism, and insulin resistance. Typically, the patients will complain of skeletal muscle weakness (often limb girdle) and will have a positive family history. Consider this disease in a patient who presents as an adult with symptoms of muscle dystrophy. These patients should be referred to a neurologist who can make the diagnosis using genetic tests. Treatment is only supportive.

NEUROMA

Morton neuroma (or Morton metatarsalgia) is a fairly common disease of the foot in which the patient has metatarsal pain. Generally it is diagnosed with MRI or ultrasound, which shows a small intrametatarsal ovoid mass. Differential diagnosis includes a metatarsal stress fracture. Treatment is surgical excision.

DEMYELINATING DISEASES

MULTIPLE SCLEROSIS

Overview

Multiple sclerosis (MS; know all the following!) is a demyelinating disease of the central nervous system that usually begins between the ages of 20 and 30. Women are affected more often than men (about 2:1). The incidence is higher in northern latitudes, possibly because of reduced sun exposure. It has recently been recognized that vitamin D may have an important role as a modifiable environmental risk factor.

The disease process is thought to be autoimmune, although no specific antibodies have been found, and the disease does not predictably respond to immunomodulators. Infections as an etiology haven't been excluded from theory.

The neurological symptoms depend on the region of brain that is affected. There are 2 types of MS:

• Relapsing-remitting (RLRM)
• Chronic progressive

The relapsing-remitting type (normal between spells) can slowly transform into the progressive type (progresses from onset). Indeed, although 85% of cases are initially RLRM, after several years, most have transformed to the progressive type.

Clinical Manifestations of MS

Paroxysmal symptoms make up the usual course of early disease (except in chronic progressive cases).

Think MS when you see relapses of the following:

• **Optic neuritis** (ON) is the most common presentation of MS eye disease, the first manifestation in about 15% of patients, and occurs at some time in 50% of all MS patients. It presents as a rapid loss of vision in one or both eyes, often accompanied by slight pain, especially on eye movement. The vision loss is usually central. With unilateral involvement, the Marcus-Gunn pupil, or afferent papillary defect, is typically seen (light shined into the eye with optic neuritis produces less constriction of both pupils than light shined into the healthy eye). With progression, the optic disk becomes pale. More than 90% of these cases recover completely.
• **Internuclear ophthalmoplegia** (IO) is another abnormal finding often seen in MS cases. IO is caused by a lesion in the "medial longitudinal fasciculus," and, although it presents as difficulty in moving the eyes horizontally, convergence is normal. (Remember that normal convergence means the patient can turn each eye inward slightly as he follows your finger to his nose, so that they continue to see a single object.) There is adduction paresis ipsilateral to the lesion, with the deficit ranging from complete medial rectus paralysis to slight slowing of an adducting saccade. Gaze-evoked horizontal jerk nystagmus is present in the abducting eye contralateral to the eye with adduction weakness. (Remember: Adduction means "toward the midline" and abduction means "away from the midline.") When you hear of a relatively young patient being diagnosed with "internuclear ophthalmoplegia," think multiple sclerosis. In older patients, however, it is more commonly due to cerebrovascular disease.
• **Other** symptoms. Generalized fatigue, nebulous sensory abnormalities (pain, paresthesias, itching, feeling of coldness or swelling, numbness [especially of the face]), vertigo/diplopia, lower-extremity motor weakness/paralysis, ataxic gait, and bowel/bladder dysfunction.

Dementia is not a typical feature of MS, especially in the earlier stages, but substantial cognitive impairment may occur in some patients with advanced chronic progressive disease. If your patient presents with dementia and gait abnormalities, a more likely diagnosis is Parkinson disease, progressive supranuclear palsy, or normal pressure hydrocephalus.

All symptoms of MS tend to worsen in the heat, called "Uhthoff phenomenon." This is because heat increases conduction block in demyelinated pathways.

Diagnosis of MS

The diagnosis of MS is no longer based only on the history and neurologic exam. The traditional (Posner) criteria incorporated signs and symptoms indicating 2 CNS lesions separated in time and space and not caused by other CNS disease. CSF findings were also used.

The fact that MS lesions disseminate over "time and space" has been, and still is, an essential component of making the diagnosis. MS develops slowly over time with new lesions occurring in different parts of the brain, thereby causing different neurological signs and symptoms. Newer criteria include CNS imaging.

MRI has become an essential tool in the workup of MS. T1 gadolinium MRI shows the characteristic enhancement or "plaques" of patchy myelin loss (white matter disease) with 90% sensitivity. T2 weighted MRI shows MS lesions as hyperintense areas (Image 11-9). Many non-MS lesions can show up as hyperintense so the specific location where these lesions are found has diagnostic weight.

Even though MRI gives the most information, it is not diagnostic, in itself.

The current McDonald criteria consider more heavily the MRI findings and have less consideration of the CSF

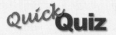

Quick Quiz

- What are the 2 common eye findings in MS?
- What findings in CSF are helpful for the diagnosis of MS? What other tests are done for the workup of MS?
- What is the treatment for an acute exacerbation of MS?
- In what clinical situation is PML likely to occur? How do these patients present?

findings than the previous (Posner) criteria. These newer criteria permit acute lesions found on MRI to be considered for the diagnosis; that is, use them to define new lesions disseminating over time and space:

- Time. A new hyperintense T2 MRI lesion more than 30 days after the initial event or T1 gadolinium enhancement more than 3 months after the initial event.
- Space (requires 3 of the following):
  ○ At least 1 T1 gadolinium-enhancing lesion or 9 T2 hyperintense lesions
  ○ At least 1 infratentorial lesion
  ○ At least 1 juxtacortical lesion
  ○ At least 3 periventricular lesions

Consider MRI of the cord in addition, especially if brain imaging doesn't reveal plaques and the patient's presentation is very suspicious for MS. The diagnostic criteria equate certain cord lesions to certain brain lesions.

MRI is also essential to rule out conditions that could mimic MS. White matter disease due to ischemia (elderly) and vasculitis both have a very different pattern of distribution from that seen with MS.

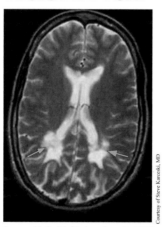

Image 11-9: Multiple sclerosis MRI

Courtesy of Steve Karceski, MD

CSF analysis helps to confirm the diagnosis. IgG immunoglobulins to myelin can be found in the cerebrospinal fluid (when these globulins are examined using electrophoresis, a few "bands" appear; thus the term oligoclonal bands). 90% of MS patients have increased IgG and oligoclonal IgG bands in the CSF. CSF protein and cell count is usually normal—on occasion, a small CSF lymphocytosis may be present, but should be no more than 50 cells/mm³.

Evoked action potentials (visual, brainstem auditory, and somatosensory-evoked potentials) can help to establish the diagnosis of MS by identifying a clinically silent second lesion.

So, again, the workup for MS now includes an MRI, a lumbar puncture, and evoked potentials. Ultimately, the diagnosis is made using a combination of clinical history, physical exam, laboratory, and imaging data.

Treatment of MS

There is no cure for MS. Treatment has now become very specialized by neurologists. As a result, general internists are expected to know that the treatment of acute exacerbations is high-dose corticosteroids (as opposed to the myriad treatment options for both intermittent and progressive disease). Glucocorticoids may shorten the duration of exacerbations but do not alter the natural history of MS. Methylprednisolone, 1 gm/day for 7 days, can be followed by a rapid prednisone taper. Some cases can be treated orally. Parenteral corticosteroids are the treatment for optic neuritis.

Other drugs used to treat chronic MS are immunomodulators (beta-interferons and monoclonal antibodies), antineoplastic drugs, and a synthetic amino acid polymer.

PROGRESSIVE MULTIFOCAL LEUKOENCEPHALOPATHY (PML)

PML (affects white matter only) is a progressive demyelination seen in patients with severe T-cell immunodeficiencies, especially HIV/AIDS patients with CD4 counts < 200 cells/mm³ that is caused by the JC virus. It is also seen in patients treated with chronic steroids or monoclonal antibodies.

An example of the monoclonal antibodies is natalizumab, used in the treatment of MS and moderate-to-severe Crohn disease. Natalizumab is an antibody to the VLA-4 antigen expressed on activated T cells and monocytes. Most cases of PML of this type have occurred with the combination of natalizumab and other immunomodulators.

The classic presentation for PML is a rapid cognitive impairment associated with motor deficits, aphasias, ataxia, and visual field defects (manifestations are variable depending on what parts of the brain/cord are affected).

Diagnose with brain biopsy. Finding JC virus by PCR in spinal fluid is supportive, although sensitivity of the PCR analysis decreases as the immune system is reconstituted on ART. ART has improved mortality in patients with PML, but many patients have persistent neurologic deficits because the nerves are unable to re-myelinate.

CENTRAL PONTINE MYELINOLYSIS

Central pontine myelinolysis (osmotic demyelination syndrome) occurs in patients with severe hyponatremia that is corrected too quickly with hypertonic saline. There is a progressively higher risk that is directly correlated with how long the patient had been hyponatremic before correction is started, how low the sodium concentration was, and how rapid the infusion of hypertonic saline is.

These patients may present with quadriparesis, mutism, pseudobulbar palsy, swallowing dysfunction, and/or locked-in syndrome. See hyponatremia in the Nephrology section for more.

MOVEMENT DISORDERS

PARKINSONISM

Parkinsonism (secondary Parkinson's, Parkinson syndrome; know this topic well) is a neurological syndrome with the characteristic set of 4 motor features (the 4 Rs).

Signs and symptoms of parkinsonism have 4 major characteristics:

- Resting tremor
- Rigidity and flexed posture
- Retarded movement (bradykinesia and hypokinesia)
- Loss of postural Reflexes

Resting tremors at a rate of 4–5 Hz (cycles per second) occur in the distal extremities. Tremor is usually the first symptom noticed. Sometimes the tremor is present with use, with dramatic worsening at rest.

Patients with parkinsonism have diffuse increased muscle tone, which, combined with the tremor, causes the "cogwheeling" seen with passive range of motion of the limbs. The flexed posture may include the entire body. The spine, elbows, hips, and knees ultimately may become flexed. The classic hand position is flexed MCP joints with straight IP joints.

Hypokinesia/bradykinesia is the primary feature. With hypokinesia, the patient has decreased amplitude of voluntary movements—especially with repetitive tasks. This may manifest as micrographia (progressive reduction in amplitude of writing). Bradykinesia is difficulty initiating movement, slowness of movement, and decrease or loss of spontaneous movement (masked facies, tendency to sit motionless, decreased blinking).

Loss of postural reflexes causes the festinating gait and eventually causes falls and then inability to stand without assistance. Festinating gait is when the patient walks progressively faster to remain under the forward center of gravity caused by truncal flexion.

There are many causes of parkinsonism. These range from Parkinson disease, to drugs, toxins, metabolic disease, infections, repeated head trauma, and vascular.

The most common cause of parkinsonism is Parkinson disease (PD; discussed next).

Many drugs can cause secondary Parkinson's. The usual culprits are:

- Dopamine-depleting drugs (e.g., reserpine)
- Dopamine antagonists such as phenothiazines or butyrophenones
- Antiemetics such as metoclopramide

Drug-induced parkinsonism is typically much more symmetric than PD.

Common toxins: Carbon monoxide and organic solvents. Repeated head trauma can also cause parkinsonism. Parkinsonism also occurs in some forms of Huntington disease (rigid form), frontotemporal dementia, and spinocerebellar ataxia.

PARKINSON DISEASE

Diagnosis

Parkinson disease (PD; know!) is a clinical diagnosis. Diagnosis is especially important and often missed in the early stages. Look for any combination of the 4 Rs of parkinsonism. Rule out causes of secondary parkinsonism. Rule out other neurodegenerative disorders. Rule out progressive supranuclear palsy (PSP; see next).

The motor features of Parkinson disease are caused by a dropout of dopamine-producing cells in the substantia nigra of the midbrain. In a normally functioning brain, the nigrostriatal neurons produce dopamine. This dopamine is released in the basal ganglia, where it has a complex effect on the motor system, facilitating voluntary movement. When there is a decrease in dopamine from deterioration of the substantia nigra, the motor symptoms of PD emerge. For reasons that are not known, symptoms always start on one side of the body and spread to the other side after a few years.

Treatment

Overview

As with MS, treatment for PD is very specialized. Focus on diagnosis, major treatments, and side effects of treatment.

Staying active and exercising are important goals that keep patients independent as long as possible.

Drugs that stimulate the dopamine system are the mainstay of therapy to treat symptoms:

- Levodopa plus carbidopa, with or without the catechol-O-methyl-transferase (COMT) inhibitor entacapone (Comtan®) or tolcapone (Tasmar®)
- Non-ergot direct dopamine receptor agonists
  ○ Ropinirole (Requip®) and pramipexole (Mirapex®)
- Amantadine
- Anticholinergics

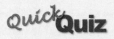

- What is the cause of central pontine myelinolysis?
- Name the 4 Rs of parkinsonism.
- What are 3 classes of drugs that are common causes of secondary parkinsonism?
- When is L-Dopa + carbidopa added to the treatment?
- What is the classic eye finding with progressive supranuclear palsy?

- Monoamine-oxidase (MAO)-B inhibitors
  - Selegiline and rasagiline

Mild

Mild symptoms, especially tremor, may respond to anticholinergics such as amantadine, benztropine (Cogentin®), and trihexyphenidyl. Anticholinergics can cause altered mental status, including psychosis, especially in patients > 70 years old and in individuals with cognitive impairment. Tricyclics, which have some anticholinergic properties, may be considered in select patients for initial therapy, as long as cognition is intact.

Treatment of Mild-to-Moderate PD

Dopamine agonists (ropinirole and pramipexole) can be useful as monotherapy for mild-to-moderate PD, but 60% of patients will require adjunctive L-dopa after 4 years.

Know that these dopa agonists are associated with impulse problems causing hypersexuality, impulse shopping, and gambling.

The MAO-B inhibitor selegiline delays the need for L-dopa in patients with mild PD by approximately 9 months. There is some evidence now that rasagiline may also slow decompensation in early Parkinson disease. To date, however, no treatment for PD has been proven to be "neuroprotective."

Special note on serotonin syndrome (serotonin toxicity): Know that combining selegiline and tricyclics or SSRIs can potentially cause the serotonin syndrome. This problem is caused by excessive serotonergic activation of both CNS and peripheral receptors. Signs and symptoms include cognitive impairment ranging from confusions to hallucinations to coma; autonomic effects such as hyperthermia, tachycardia, shivering, sweating; and somatic effects such as hyperreflexia and clonus, twitching, and tremors. Symptoms can be mild to rapidly fatal, depending on the amount of overstimulation.

Treatment of Severe PD

More severe symptoms are usually treated with L-dopa + carbidopa. L-dopa acts as a precursor for dopamine synthesis in the basal ganglia. The carbidopa blocks conversion of L-dopa to dopamine in the periphery, a desirable effect because peripheral dopamine does not cross the blood-brain barrier. Additionally, peripheral dopamine causes side effects such as postural hypotension and nausea. Carbidopa does not help with the central side effects of L-dopa that emerge after several years.

Note that L-dopa absorption may be reduced by dietary protein.

Although L-dopa is the most effective drug for PD, its use is withheld as long as possible, especially in younger patients, to delay the onset of complications that are common with chronic use—especially psychosis, dyskinesias, and motor fluctuations (see below).

Direct dopamine receptor agonists (ropinirole and pramipexole) and COMT inhibitors (entacapone or tolcapone) are added to reduce the overall daily dose of L-dopa, to even out the serum levels of this drug, and to provide more continuous dopamine receptor stimulation.

The older dopamine agonists (bromocriptine, cabergoline, and pergolide) may have ergot-related adverse effects, including a risk of valvular heart disease. Cabergoline should not be used to treat Parkinson's patients; it remains available for treatment of prolactinomas.

Neural tissue transplants may result in "runaway dyskinesias" and are currently not recommended for PD.

Complications of PD therapy include the following:

- End-of-dose "wearing off" effects (due to short half-life of L-dopa).
- Unpredictable "on-off" fluctuations that are characterized by unpredictable loss of treatment effect and dyskinesias (50% of patients after 3–5 years).
- Psychiatric symptoms develop in 30% of patients treated with L-dopa. These symptoms include agitation, confusion, depression, and hallucinations. Older patients with cognitive impairment are especially at risk.

"Drug holiday" is typically no longer used to treat complications of long-term L-dopa use because it carries a low risk of serious complications such as aspiration pneumonia, pulmonary embolism, venous thrombosis, and depression.

PROGRESSIVE SUPRANUCLEAR PALSY

Progressive supranuclear palsy (PSP) is similar to Parkinson disease in that patients have bradykinesia, abnormal gait, increased muscle tone, and later develop dementia. These patients have an erect posture with hyperextension of the neck, especially later in the course

NEUROLOGY

of the disease. They usually do not have a tremor. Within 2 years, the patients develop the classic symptom of a vertical ophthalmoplegia, typically with initial impairment of downgaze, progressing to complete ophthalmoplegia in all directions. Subsequently, the patients have trouble reading, eating, and walking down stairs. Within another 2–3 years, the patients may be unable to walk because of marked imbalance. There is no specific treatment.

TREMORS

Action tremors occur with intentional movement and disappear at rest. They have 2 main causes:

- Exaggerated physiologic tremor
- Essential tremor

The rate of the normal physiologic tremor is 9 Hz. It is aggravated by anxiety, hyperthyroidism, and certain drugs (theophylline, β-agonists, caffeine). Essential tremor has a similar frequency (8–10 Hz) and is often familial. In the latter case, it seems to be transmitted as an autosomal dominant trait, with variation in age at onset and severity. Essential tremor is usually benign but sometimes results in functional disability. It is typically decreased transiently by drinking alcohol (you can often diagnose the tremor this way; patients will tell you it gets better after a glass of wine). Propranolol and primidone are first-line drugs and may be at least partially effective in half of patients; gabapentin and topiramate may also help to suppress the tremor. In severe cases, botulinum toxin and deep-brain stimulation surgery can be tried.

TARDIVE DYSKINESIA

Tardive dyskinesia is usually a result of long-term antipsychotic drug use. The only way to be certain to avoid tardive is to keep patients off chronic antipsychotics, but this cannot be accomplished in many patients with chronic psychosis.

Tardive dyskinesia consists of chorea of the lips, tongue, face, and neck—and occasionally affects the limbs.

The "atypical antipsychotics" (2nd generation drugs), such as clozapine and quetiapine fumarate (Seroquel®), may be less likely to cause tardive. Know that clozapine can cause bone marrow toxicity.

Clonazepam is a useful benzodiazepine for patients with mild tardive and anxiety. Severe cases can be treated with botulinum toxin. Deep-brain stimulation surgery can be used in the most severe cases that require continued use of antipsychotic drugs.

OTHER MOVEMENT DISORDERS

Neuroleptic Malignant Syndrome

Neuroleptic malignant syndrome is an unusual response to antipsychotics (both "typical" and "atypical" antipsychotics), resulting in fever, rigidity, autonomic instability, and altered mental status, with a risk of rhabdomyolysis-induced renal failure. Occasionally, other drugs can do it also, such as metoclopramide and promethazine. Labs often show leukocytosis, electrolyte disturbances, and elevated CK levels.

Know that Parkinson patients who acutely discontinue their dopa therapy (or dose reduce) can develop this syndrome.

Treatment consists of immediate discontinuation of any offending drug; use of a direct dopamine agonist such as bromocriptine, amantadine, or dantrolene; and supportive therapy, including adequate hydration and scrupulous pulmonary toilet. If rigidity is sufficient to affect ventilation, the patient should be sedated and paralyzed. Patients who require neuroleptics may or may not have recurrence of neuroleptic malignant syndrome if the drugs are restarted.

Hemifacial Spasm

Hemifacial spasm is a motor analog to trigeminal neuralgia (tic douloureux). 80% of patients have a tortuous, dilated basilar artery that irritates the facial nerve!

Best treatment is botulinum injections.

Gilles de la Tourette

Gilles de la Tourette is a movement disorder characterized by motor and/or vocal tics that usually begins between 2 and 15 years of age. Many patients have comorbid attention-deficit hyperactivity disorder (ADHD), obsessive-compulsive disorder, learning disorders, or conduct disorders.

Diagnosis is clinical and requires observation of vocal tics.

If the tics are severe enough to interfere with daily functioning, dopa antagonists can be used (fluphenazine, pimozide) or typical antipsychotics (haloperidol). ADHD with tics can be treated with methylphenidate—newer data show that the drug does not exacerbate tics, as we previously thought.

Focal Dystonias

Three focal dystonias commonly asked about are:

1) Oromandibular dystonia (Meige syndrome) causes incessant movement of the lower jaw.
2) Blepharospasm is bilateral, involuntary eye closure and may occur as an isolated syndrome or as part of Meige syndrome.
3) Torticollis occurs when spasms of neck and shoulder muscles turn the head to one side.

A few oral drugs may offer mild relief: benzodiazepines, baclofen, anticholinergics, and sometimes antidopaminergics. However, botulinum toxin is now the treatment of choice, providing much more reliable but temporary relief when injected directly into the affected muscles. It requires repeat injections q 2–5 months.

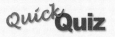

- What are the 3 main causes of unilateral blindness in the older age group?
- What is dimmimg of vision after exercise called? What disease is it seen with?
- What is a Marcus Gunn pupil? What disease is it most commonly associated with?
- What are flashes followed by decreased vision suggestive of?

MISCELLANEOUS DISORDERS

ACUTE-ONSET UNILATERAL BLINDNESS

Know all of the following and see Table 11-8 for a summary.

In older patients, acute onset of unilateral blindness is usually due to any of the following:

- Anterior ischemic optic neuropathy (AION), which may be:
  - Arteritic (secondary to giant cell arteritis)
  - Non-arteritic (less severe outcome)
- Retinal vein occlusion (2nd to diabetic retinopathy as a cause of vision loss from retinal vascular disease)
- Retinal artery occlusion (from thrombus or from emboli from the carotid artery or heart)

In the younger patient, think optic neuritis, but sometimes it can be from migraine. Migraine-induced blindness usually resolves rapidly, whereas blindness due to any of the other mentioned causes is prolonged or permanent.

Ischemic optic neuropathy, optic neuritis, and papilledema all can present with swollen discs with fundal splinter hemorrhages. Remember that temporal (giant cell) arteritis also causes diplopia and jaw claudication.

"Malingering" as a cause of blindness (mono/bi) can be ruled out with evoked action potentials.

DIPLOPIA

Weak or paralyzed eye muscles cause "ophthalmoplegia" and manifest as diplopia. It can be a result of disease in the muscle itself or disease in the nerve that stimulates the muscle.

A reminder of diseases that may present with diplopia. We have covered most of these separately:

- 3rd and 6th nerve palsies
- Myasthenia
- Graves disease
- Wernicke encephalopathy
- Miller Fisher variant of GBS
- Botulism
- Tick paralysis
- Infections/masses that affect the cavernous sinus

If you see diplopia with pain:

- Think disease in the eyeball if pain is localized in the eye.
- Think myopathy or orbital processes if pain is present with movement of the eye. Influenza is a classic cause of orbital myopathy.

Optic neuritis may also cause pain on eye movement but it does not cause diplopia!

VISUAL FIELD DEFECTS

Scotomas

Scotomas are alterations in an isolated area of the visual field with loss or dimness of vision. Do a complete ophthalmologic exam on any patient with any type of scotoma.

Acephalic migraine (migraine without headache) can cause "fortification scotomas" that constantly change in size and may be bilateral.

Moore's lightning streaks occur in older patients upon entering a darkened area. They are caused by the vitreous pulling on the retina; they are benign.

Retinal detachment causes flashes followed by decreased vision (from blood) or increased floaters.

		Table 11-8: Causes of Acute Unilateral Blindness			
Age	**Disease**	**Etiology**	**Clinical Course**	**Exam**	**Outcome**
Older (> 50)	Anterior ischemic optic neuropathy	< 60: atherosclerosis > 60: giant cell arteritis	Nonprogressive	Optic disk infarction	From normal to complete blindness
	Central retinal vein occlusion	Hypotension; diabetes	Nonprogressive	Hemorrhagic retinopathy	Usually some visual impairment
	Central retinal artery occlusion	Embolic or thrombotic	Nonprogressive	Cherry red spot	Only ~ 25% maintain useful vision
Younger (< 40)	Optic neuritis	Multiple sclerosis	Progressive (hours to days)	Marcus Gunn pupil; optic disc pallor	90% recover completely
	Migraine	Neurovascular	Resolves rapidly	Normal	Normal vision

NEUROLOGY

Bitemporal Hemianopsia

Bitemporal hemianopsia is the term for blindness in the lateral half of both visual fields. It has several causes:

- Pituitary adenomas (this is the one we all remember)
- Craniopharyngioma
- Meningioma
- Aneurysm of the circle of Willis
- Sarcoidosis (rare)
- Metastatic carcinoma (rare)

REFLEX SYMPATHETIC DYSTROPHY

Reflex sympathetic dystrophy causes pain, swelling, dysesthesias, and vasomotor instability in an extremity after a traumatic injury.

NARCOLEPSY

Narcolepsy is caused by a selective loss of hypocretin in the hypothalamus, the etiology of which is currently unknown.

More than 85% of Caucasian and Japanese patients with narcolepsy-cataplexy syndrome have a specific HLA haplotype that includes HLA-DR1501 (formerly called DR15 or DR2) and HLA-DQB1-0602 (formerly DQ1 or DQ6).

Narcolepsy quartet:

1) Narcolepsy
2) Cataplexy (3/4 of patients! With excitement, limbs become flaccid)
3) Hypnagogic hallucinations (occur as patient falls asleep)
4) Sleep paralysis (on waking)

Narcolepsy is treated with modafinil (a non-amphetamine drug) or stimulants such as methylphenidate or methamphetamine (many side effects and addictive potential). Cataplexy is treated with tricyclics (imipramine, clomipramine, or protriptyline) or the serotonin reuptake inhibitors (e.g. venlafaxine or fluoxetine).

MedStudy®

IM
INTERNAL MEDICINE REVIEW
CORE CURRICULUM

14th EDITION

Authored by Robert A. Hannaman, MD
with J. Thomas Cross, Jr., MD, MPH, FACP

DERMATOLOGY

DERMATOLOGY

Many thanks to Dermatology Advisor:

Margery Atkins Scott, MD
Clinical Professor of Dermatology
Department of Dermatology
Eastern Virginia Medical School
Norfolk, VA

Table of Contents
Dermatology

COMMON SKIN PROBLEMS

ATOPIC DERMATITIS

Atopic dermatitis (AD) (Image 12-1) has three age-group categories: infant (0–2 years), childhood (2–12 years), and adult (> 12 years; least common). 85% of all cases start at < 5 years of age. Each stage may be a continuation of the previous stage or may be a new finding. It is multifactorial, occasionally with increased IgE. Usually, there is a family history of asthma and/or rhinitis; however, recent studies have called this association into question. Patients have a decreased itching threshold and dry skin. They develop pruritic skin rashes, initially erythematous, edematous patches found on the head and neck. Extensor surfaces tend to be involved in infants; in children and adults, involvement is more often flexural. These may crust and then "weep," at least partly from scratching.

Hydration, water-trapping agents, moderate-strength topical corticosteroids, and occasional systemic immunosuppressants are the mainstay of treatment for AD, as well as other immunosuppressants and ultraviolet radiation.

Tacrolimus (Protopic®) and pimecrolimus (Elidel®) are new topical immunosuppressants that are effective alternatives to topical corticosteroids. Since these don't cause skin atrophy, they are especially good for facial lesions. There is a potential risk of cancer, so these agents are second-line for intermittent treatment of atopic dermatitis. They are not to be used on children < 2 years or anybody with weakened immune systems.

Oral cyclosporine, azathioprine, or methotrexate is used for severe AD that does not respond to conservative therapy.

Antigens, such as *S. aureus* or dust mites, and stress can exacerbate AD. Because of decreased skin defenses, AD patients tend to get chronic bacterial and fungal skin colonization and infections. Occasionally, oral antibiotics are given to decrease colonization of *S. aureus* and thus improve the course of the disease.

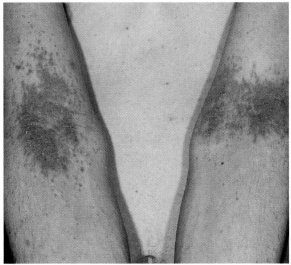

Image 12-1: Antecubital fossa with atopic dermatitis

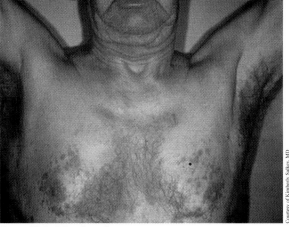

Image 12-2: Seborrheic dermatitis

SEBORRHEA

Seborrheic dermatitis manifests as erythema and has a greasy scale (Image 12-2). It especially involves the scalp (dandruff), eyebrows, paranasal area, and external auditory canal. There is a strong association with *Malassezia furfur*, but it is unknown if this fungus is a cause or result of the dermatitis.

Seborrheic dermatitis is common in patients with HIV/AIDS and Parkinson disease.

Treatment of seborrheic dermatitis: frequent washing and an antiproliferative shampoo for the dandruff. The active ingredients in antiproliferative shampoos are selenium sulfide, zinc pyrithione, salicylic acid, or tar. The antimicrobial shampoos include ketoconazole or ciclopirox, and some are formulated with antiproliferative agents as well.

Use low-potency topical corticosteroids or ketoconazole cream for skin disease.

INTERTRIGO

Intertrigo is an irritant dermatitis found in the macerated skin folds of obese patients. It commonly is due to *Candida*.

Treat with topical antifungals and drying agents (antifungal powders, aluminum sulfate products, corn starch). Avoid the use of talcum powder in the genital area of women because of the increased risk of ovarian cancer.

CONTACT DERMATITIS

Contact dermatitis can be caused by a chemical irritant (80% of contact dermatitis is due to irritants), or it can be of allergic origin (Image 12-3). The most common irritants are soapy water, rubbing alcohol, and common household cleaners. The allergic type is due

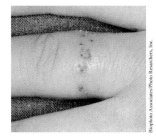

Image 12-3: Contact dermatitis caused by ring with nickel

DERMATOLOGY

to a delayed hypersensitivity reaction in the skin. Patients can become sensitized to the antigen with one or many exposures. After sensitization and upon re-exposure, the skin will develop a pruritic lesion in 1/2 to 2 days. Most common allergens are nickel, chromium, neomycin, and oleoresin urushiol (poison oak, poison ivy, and poison sumac). Treatment is cool compresses, Burow's solution (aluminum acetate dissolved in water, 1:40), and topical corticosteroids. If severe or involves the face, give systemic corticosteroids.

ACNE

Acne Vulgaris

The clinical manifestations of acne vulgaris are:

- Open and closed comedones
- Papules
- Pustules
- Cystic lesions
- Ice-pick scars
- Postinflammatory hyperpigmentation

Comedonal acne is noninflammatory acne, which develops in early adolescence.

Inflammatory acne is due to *Propionibacterium acnes* within the follicle. Acne severity is genetic and hormonal, with an imbalance between estrogens and androgens. However, contrary to popular belief, most patients with acne do not overproduce androgens; likely the sebaceous glands are locally hyperresponsive to androgens (hence the genetic predisposition for many).

Factors that may exacerbate acne include cosmetics, oils, repetitive mechanical trauma (scrubbing), clothing (turtlenecks, bra straps, and sports helmets), humidity, and heavy sweating. Diet is controversial; some studies have shown an association with milk intake (exacerbating) and low-glycemic diets (ameliorating). Stress appears to worsen acne severity.

Acne vulgaris differs from rosacea by the presence of comedones (seen in acne vulgaris) and the lack of telangiectasia (not seen in acne vulgaris). See Image 12-4 through Image 12-6.

Note that acne is a common manifestation of increased androgens; it is often an external manifestation of polycystic ovary syndrome (PCO) in women. But having acne is not usually associated with increased androgens. PCO occurs in 5–10% of women, and about 1/3 of women with acne have PCO.

Treatment of acne vulgaris:

Comedonal (noninflammatory) acne: Topical retinoids are drugs of choice for comedonal acne. These include adapalene, tretinoin, and tazarotene (note: Tazarotene [Tazorac®] is contraindicated in pregnancy!).

Side effects are mainly skin irritation and photosensitivity. Other agents for comedonal acne include topical salicylic acid, azelaic acid, and glycolic acid; all 3 have anticomedonal activity.

Mild inflammatory acne (Image 12-4): Benzoyl peroxide in combination with topical erythromycin or clindamycin is used to treat the *P. acnes* of inflammatory acne. The combination therapy decreases development of resistance, and commercial preparations are available that have both products. Topical retinoids are also useful in combination. Topical dapsone, an effective antimicrobial agent, was initially approved by the FDA in 1955; in 2009, it was remarketed with the trade name Aczone®.

Moderate-to-severe inflammatory acne (Image 12-5): This usually requires oral antibiotics in addition to the above topical therapy. The oral antibiotics used are tetracycline, doxycycline, minocycline, and erythromycin. TMP/SMX is occasionally used. If oral isotretinoin is used, all other acne treatments should be stopped.

Isotretinoin (Amnesteem®, Claravis®, Sotret®; 1.0 mg/kg/d) is highly effective in resistant cases but is also a powerful teratogen. The use of isotretinoin is restricted to physicians who have registered with the electronic FDA system (called the "iPLEDGE program") and requires multiple steps in order to prescribe (2 pregnancy tests, 2 forms of birth control, etc.). Serious side effects include pseudotumor cerebri (especially if used with tetracyclines), depression and psychosis, pancreatitis, marked hypertriglyceridemia, hearing loss, night vision loss, and skeletal abnormalities.

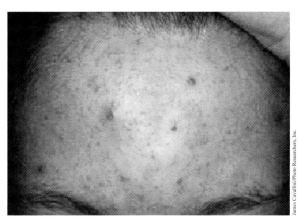

Image 12-4: Mild inflammatory acne

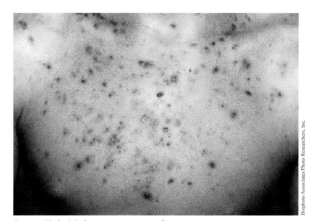

Image 12-5: Moderate-to-severe inflammatory acne

DERMATOLOGY

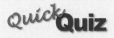

Quick Quiz

- What is seborrhea?
- What is intertrigo?
- Contact dermatitis is an example of what type of hypersensitivity reaction?
- What are the serious side effects of isotretinoin?
- What finding on the oral mucosa can be seen with measles? Describe and name the finding.
- What viral disease causes oral leukoplakia?

Hormonal therapy with oral contraceptives is effective for women with excessive androgen production, particularly PCO. Spironolactone is also used for hormonal therapy.

Acne Rosacea

Acne rosacea (Image 12-6) occurs in mostly middle-aged patients and presents with acne-like lesions, erythema, and telangiectasias on the central face. Even before the lesions, the patients may have a flushing reaction to various stimuli (e.g., alcohol, stress). Once the rosacea manifests, the flush may become permanent. Treatment is usually tetracycline, topical metronidazole, azelaic acid, or sulfur/sulfacetamide preparations. Rhinophyma (big nose) also occurs and may require surgical therapy.

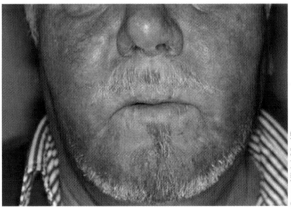

Image 12-6: Acne rosacea

HIDRADENITIS

Hidradenitis suppurativa (acne inversa) is a chronic inflammatory scarring process involving apocrine gland-bearing areas (Image 12-7). The problem starts with follicular keratinization and apocrinitis, which plug the apocrine duct, resulting in dilation of the duct and subsequent inflammation of adjacent apocrine glands (particularly glands in the axilla and groin areas). This disease occurs in both sexes—women tend to have more axillary and vulvar involvement while perianal involvement is more common in men.

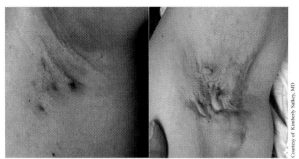

Image 12-7: Hidradenitis suppurativa; mild vs. severe

The disease process can range from mild to severe (induration, scarring, pitting, and draining abscesses).

Treatment for hidradenitis is often ineffective. Avoid deodorants (antiperspirants okay); tight, synthetic clothing; and prolonged exposure to hot, humid environments. Treat acute infections with incision, drainage, and packing. Try tetracycline or erythromycin, then a topical antibiotic for prophylaxis. Oral contraceptives may be used in women. Give zinc gluconate to prevent lesions. Newer therapies include biologics, which have produced some success. Surgical excision is the only definitive therapy for severe cases.

MOUTH FINDINGS

Know all of these!

Hyperpigmented gingiva is seen in Addison disease.

Koplik spots (Image 12-8) are small white vesicles on an erythematous base, which are found on the palate in patients with measles. These usually precede the skin lesions by several days.

Oral hairy leukoplakia (Image 12-9) most commonly occurs in patients with HIV/AIDS. It appears as areas of ribbed whiteness along the sides of the tongue. This is due to Epstein-Barr virus in the superficial layers of the tongue's squamous epithelium.

Peutz-Jeghers syndrome (multiple intestinal hamartomatous polyps) should be ruled out in patients with melanotic pigmentation (lentigines) on the lips and buccal mucosa.

Beefy red tongue and angular cheilitis are associated with glucagonomas—discussed under "Skin Cancer and Skin Findings" on page 12-11.

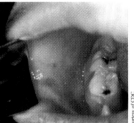

Image 12-8: Koplik spots

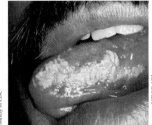

Image 12-9: Oral hairy leukoplakia

Macroglossia (big tongue) is associated with multiple myeloma, primary amyloidosis, lymphoma, hemangioma, acromegaly, and Down syndrome.

White lesions: Candidiasis, hairy leukoplakia (AIDS), lichen planus. Lichen planus also causes ulceration and lace-like patches.

"Geographic" tongue has the appearance of migratory denuded red patches. It is asymptomatic and benign (Image 12-10).

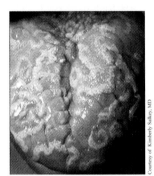

Image 12-10: Geographic tongue

"Strawberry" tongue is associated with scarlet fever, toxic shock syndrome, and Kawasaki disease (mucocutaneous lymph node syndrome; children usually).

"Bald" tongue is an atrophy of the tongue associated with pellagra, iron deficiency anemia, pernicious anemia, and xerostomia (salivary gland problems as seen in Sjögren syndrome, lymphoma, mumps, and sarcoidosis; occasionally idiopathic).

CUTANEOUS DRUG REACTIONS

The following are the most frequent drug-associated skin changes.

Penicillin (PCN):
- Immediate hypersensitivity reaction; anaphylaxis (IgE)
- Delayed hypersensitivity reaction; immune complex reaction, such as vasculitis or morbilliform eruption

Tetracycline: Photosensitivity

NSAIDs: Urticaria/angioedema in 1%, asthma in 0.5%, and may cause photosensitivity or toxic epidermal necrolysis (TEN).

Phenytoin:
- Hypersensitivity syndrome: purpura, facial edema, lymphadenopathy, and hepatitis
- Various skin reactions, including erythema multiforme
- Hypertrophied gums

Corticosteroids: Skin changes, including striae, atrophy, telangiectasia, pigmentary changes, and acne-like lesions.

Warfarin: Necrotic patches (necrosis) of skin appearing 3–10 days after starting warfarin.

Radiocontrast dye: This can cause urticaria/erythema (1/15), and anaphylaxis (1/1,000). There is a 30% repeat reaction incidence in someone with a previous reaction to contrast dye. The repeat reaction can be very serious. Prophylaxis with diphenhydramine and corticosteroids (start 1–2 days prior) will decrease this reaction 10-fold.

ACE inhibitors: Angioedema occurs in only 0.5% of patients treated with an ACE inhibitor, but because such a large number of patients receive the drug, it is one of the most common causes of isolated angioedema.

INFLAMMATORY SKIN DISORDERS

NOTE

Many of the disorders described here are presented in more detail in the Rheumatology section.

PSORIASIS

Overview

Psoriasis is a response triggered by T lymphocytes in the skin.

Types of Psoriasis

Plaque psoriasis is the most common type (Image 12-11). It presents in young adults with well-defined, stable, slow-growing, non-pruritic, erythematous skin lesions with distinctive mica-like (silvery) scales. It is usually symmetric and occurs on extensor surfaces of the knees and elbows, the sacral area, and the scalp.

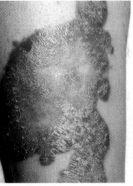

Image 12-11: Plaque psoriasis

Koebner phenomenon (outbreak in the area of trauma) is common. See the Rheumatology section for psoriatic arthritis.

Guttate (eruptive) psoriasis is an abrupt eruption of multiple small lesions, which usually occurs on the trunk of children or young adults with no previous history of psoriasis. There is a strong association with upper respiratory infections and group A beta-hemolytic strep.

Flexural (inverse) psoriasis affects skinfold areas. Called inverse because it is not on the extensor surfaces.

There are 2 especially severe types of psoriasis:

1) Erythrodermic psoriasis
2) Pustular psoriasis

Erythrodermic psoriasis is an exfoliative reaction in which the entire surface of the skin becomes red, warm, and scaly; and, the patient is unable to control body temperature (hypo/hyperthermia is common). Dehydration, hypoalbuminemia, and anemia of chronic disease are common sequelae. The erythroderma and psoriasis of any type are often precipitated/exacerbated by sunburn, infection (virus, strep pharyngitis), and drugs (especially antimalarials, gold, lithium, and beta-blockers). Alcohol and cancer do not exacerbate psoriasis. Treatment can include acitretin (Soriatane®), cyclosporine, biologics, and sometimes methotrexate.

Pustular psoriasis has many small pustules, often coalescing to form "psoriatic lakes of pus." 2 forms:

1) The localized form affects only the palms and soles. It is associated with DIP joint arthritis.
2) The rare, generalized form (von Zumbusch type) is the most severe form of psoriasis and may occur with the erythrodermic type.

Nail Changes

The most specific nail finding is an "oil slick" (glycoprotein) deposition in nails. "Ice-pick" pitting of the nails is common. These pits will usually be in small groups on the nail. Thickened nails and onycholysis (separation of distal nail from the nail bed) are also common in psoriasis (Image 12-12). Having pitted nails in association with onycholysis is fairly specific for psoriasis and psoriatic arthritis.

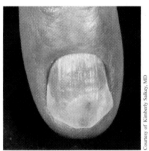

Image 12-12: Pitted nail with onycholysis

Drugs Used to Treat Psoriasis

(Know these.)

Topical corticosteroids: Plaques are usually treated with topical corticosteroids; oral agents may actually worsen the disease.

Tar is time-honored and often still used in a compounded preparation with a corticosteroid. Tar preparations stain clothes but are well tolerated.

Calcineurin inhibitors: Topical tacrolimus (Protopic®) and topical pimecrolimus (Elidel®). Often used for facial and intertriginous areas when high-potency steroids should be avoided. Be aware of the FDA boxed warning for a potential increased risk of lymphoma and skin malignancy.

Retinoids (vitamin A derivatives):
- Tazarotene gel (Tazorac®, Avage®, topical retinoids) compares well with topical steroids.
- Acitretin (Soriatane®), a second-generation oral retinoid, is used for the severe forms of all types. Do not use in women with child-bearing potential.

Vitamin D_3 analog:
- Calcipotriene (Dovonex®, a synthetic vitamin D_3 analog) compares well with topical steroids.
- Calcitriol (Vectical®, a synthetic vitamin D_3 analog in an ointment base).

Immunosuppressants:
- Methotrexate
- Cyclosporine
- Azathioprine

Biologic immunomodulators:

These are new, effective treatments for psoriasis:
- T-cell memory effector inhibitor: alefacept (Amevive®)
- TNF-alpha inhibitors: etanercept (Enbrel®), infliximab (Remicade®), adalimumab (Humira®)
- IL-12 and IL-23 blocker: ustekinumab (Stelara™)

Ultraviolet light may be added to the above treatments. UVB (290–320 nm) therapy is often used. Narrow-band UVB (311 nm) is possibly more effective than the broader spectrum treatment (few good studies) but requires more expensive equipment.

"PUVA" (oral psoralen + UVA light [320–400 nm]) is also very effective and is usually given to those who fail UVB. UVA penetrates more deeply than UVB and is less likely to burn (hence, the photosensitizing psoralen), but it is associated with increased likelihood of skin cancer, including melanoma.

Methotrexate and **cyclosporine** are commonly used for widespread psoriasis, especially with arthritis. Remember: Do not give methotrexate to patients with liver/renal disease or a history of alcohol abuse.

Again: Several drugs used to treat RA also treat psoriatic arthritis and psoriasis: cyclosporine, methotrexate, and etanercept (Enbrel®; a TNF receptor blocker).

DERMATOLOGY

Treatment of Psoriasis

Mild plaque psoriasis: Treat with hydration and water trapping agents. Use high-potency or ultra–high-potency topical corticosteroids (except for the face, axillae, and genitalia: use low-potency treatment or use topical tacrolimus or pimecrolimus), calcipotriene, or topical retinoids (tazarotene) for mild plaques.

Moderate psoriasis: Treat with high-potency topical corticosteroids, calcipotriene, topical retinoids (tazarotene), or UVB therapy.

Widespread or severe: Use a combination of UVB or PUVA, oral retinoids (acitretin), and biologic immunomodulators.

Guttate psoriasis: Treat with UVB plus or minus topical steroids. Treat any streptococcal infection!

Flexural psoriasis: Treat with low-potency topical corticosteroids or topical tacrolimus/pimecrolimus.

LUPUS

Systemic lupus erythematosus (SLE):

Malar (or butterfly) rash occurs in about half of SLE patients. Classically, this rash involves both cheeks and extends across the bridge of the nose sparing the nasolabial fold. The malar rash is erythematous and either flat or slightly edematous and often occurs after sunlight exposure (photosensitive). No scarring.

Patchy and diffuse nonscarring alopecia is common.

More on SLE in the Rheumatology section.

Discoid lupus erythematosus (DLE): Discoid lesions are erythematous and raised with slightly tight scales. They cause atrophic scarring. They usually occur on the face, scalp, and neck. Only 5–10% of DLE patients develop SLE.

SYSTEMIC SCLEROSIS

Morphea is a localized scleroderma characterized by plaques that become sclerotic with a hypopigmented center and erythematous border. It usually occurs in children or young adults. It can be just a few lesions (localized morphea) or widespread with some confluence (generalized morphea).

Diffuse systemic sclerosis (previously scleroderma) (Image 12-13) usually starts with recurrent, non-pitting edema of the face and distal extremities and involves internal organs. Sclerosis of the skin begins at the distal digits and moves proximally. Patients may develop

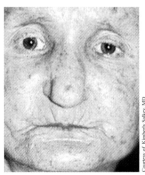
Image 12-13: Systemic sclerosis

tight, unwrinkled skin over the face, and the fingers may become tight and sausage-shaped. No nail changes, but nailfold capillary changes are commonly seen and correlate with severity of disease. No satisfactory treatment.

Limited systemic sclerosis (previously CREST) is a grouping of symptoms that has limited systemic involvement. These patients present with calcinosis cutis (small tender nodules on the fingers), Raynaud syndrome, esophageal dysmotility, sclerodactyly of the fingers, and telangiectasias.

SARCOIDOSIS

Sarcoidosis is an immune-related noncaseating granulomatous disease that often affects the lungs, lymph nodes, eyes, and skin. Skin involvement is seen in about 20% of cases. Lesions are:

• Erythema nodosum (see next). Sarcoidosis is one of the most common causes of E. nodosum. Unlike the other skin findings, this is associated with a good prognosis and shows no caseation. Do not biopsy E. nodosum in sarcoidosis for diagnosis—the histopathology will just show a panniculitis and not granulomas.
• Erythematous papules, mainly around face.
• Scar sarcoidosis presents as granulomatous changes in a healing skin wound (laceration, tattoo, etc.).
• Plaque-like lesions.

Sarcoidosis is the second-greatest mimic of other diseases (first is syphilis); it can mimic any dermatologic disease, except a vesicular eruption.

Lupus pernio is a type of sarcoidosis that has skin changes ranging from violaceous lesions on the tip of the nose and earlobes to large purple nodules/tumors on the face and fingers. It has a slow onset and almost never resolves!

The best prognosis of the sarcoid skin changes is with E. nodosum or the small papules. Treat a cutaneous sarcoid with intralesional/topical steroids, occasionally antimalarials, and methotrexate. Dapsone is ineffective.

ERYTHEMA NODOSUM

Erythema nodosum (Image 12-14) consists of red, warm, very tender nodules that usually appear on the shins. Although sarcoidosis is one of the most common causes of erythema nodosum, other causes include inflammatory bowel disease, infection (TB, streptococcal, deep fungal), and drugs (esp. oral contraceptives, sulfas, and penicillins). Worldwide, streptococcal infection is likely the most common cause of erythema nodosum. Know all of these causes!

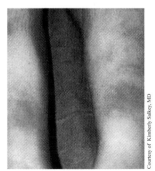
Image 12-14: Erythema nodosum

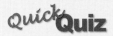

Quick Quiz

- What are the differences in treatments for mild, moderate, and severe widespread psoriasis?
- What systemic lung disease is one of the common causes of erythema nodosum? Know the other causes too!
- If you see the words "periorbital heliotropic rash," think of this!
- How does zinc deficiency manifest on the skin?

DERMATOMYOSITIS

Buzzwords: periorbital heliotropic rash (+/– periorbital edema) (Image 12-15). This is a violaceous, sometimes scaly rash in a photosensitive distribution, which looks very much like a localized allergic reaction.

Gottron papules, seen in dermatomyositis, are flat-topped, reddish-to-violet, sometimes scaling papules; sometimes, they just look like "cigarette paper" crinkling of the skin over the knuckles (MCP, PIP, and/or DIP). Gottron papules are the most specific finding with dermatomyositis. They may be described only as a "rash" or "eruption" over the knuckles (Image 12-16).

Livedo reticularis is pretty nonspecific; it is seen in dermatomyositis but also in cutaneous polyarteritis nodosa, SLE, antiphospholipid antibody syndrome, and cholesterol embolism (atheroembolism); and there is a fairly common benign idiopathic type.

Treatment is corticosteroids +/– immunomodulators. Remember: In older patients, dermatomyositis may indicate cancer (GU, GI, and respiratory are most common).

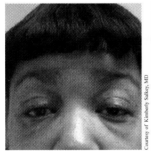
Image 12-15: Periorbital heliotropic rash

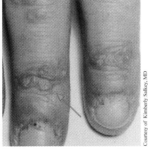
Image 12-16: Gottron papules

REACTIVE ARTHRITIS

Reactive arthritis (previously Reiter syndrome) causes pustular scaly lesions on the palms and soles (keratoderma blennorrhagicum; Image 12-17) and circinate balanitis on the penis.

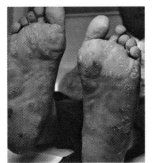
Image 12-17: Reiter syndrome keratoderma

VASCULITIS

The main cutaneous reaction with vasculitis is palpable purpura, usually starting on the legs. If a patient presents with arthralgias, abdominal pain, and palpable purpura, think Henoch-Schönlein purpura—not reactive arthritis.

PYODERMA GANGRENOSUM

Pyoderma gangrenosum is an inflammatory ulcer usually occurring on the legs (Image 12-18). It is often associated with inflammatory bowel disease. It can also occur with rheumatoid arthritis, leukemia, IgA gammopathy, and chronic active hepatitis. Although a skin biopsy is not diagnostic, it serves to exclude other causes for ulceration. Treating the colonized bacteria usually does not help. First-line treatment is prednisone.

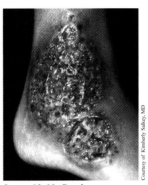
Image 12-18: Pyoderma gangrenosum

VITAMIN DEFICIENCIES

Deficiency of B12, folate, or niacin may cause diffuse hyperpigmentation, as well as hair and nail changes. Niacin deficiency results in the 3 Ds: dermatitis, diarrhea, and dementia.

Zinc deficiency causes an irritant eczematoid red rash that usually involves the nasolabial folds, extensor surfaces, and perineum/scrotum.

SKIN INFECTIONS

BACTERIAL SKIN INFECTIONS

Much of the following and all treatments are covered more fully in the Infectious Disease section.

Corynebacterium

Erythrasma is a well-defined, reddish lesion with some slight scaling. It is usually found in the axilla, groin, and toe webs. In obese women, it is seen under the breasts. Gram-positive *Corynebacterium minutissimum* is frequently isolated from the lesion (especially after it has become scaly or macerated). DDx: Fungal infection and intertrigo (an irritant dermatitis found in the skin folds of obese patients). Diagnosis: Erythrasma fluoresces bright red with the Wood's lamp. Treat with oral or topical erythromycin +/– an "-azole" antifungal cream.

Streptococcus pyogenes (group A strep)

Impetigo. Group A strep is a cause of impetigo—a skin infection confined to the epidermis. Also see *S. aureus*, below.

Ecthyma starts as an impetigo and then becomes deeper, causing shallow ulcerations.

Erysipelas is an explosive superficial infection (often caused by group A strep), confined to the dermis, that spreads quickly through skin lymphatics (Image 12-19). There is a clearly demarcated area of redness that is often palpable, indicating infection. It usually starts from a superficial abrasion, typically around the central face, with erythema and swelling.

Necrotizing fasciitis (streptococcal gangrene) has been in the media ("flesh-eating bacteria"). It is a deep, soft tissue infection involving subcutaneous fat and fascia. Unlike erysipelas, it does not have a distinct border and can be difficult to diagnose early. Also, the infection can be polymicrobial (e.g., group A strep + anaerobes). There is high mortality even with appropriate medical and surgical intervention.

Scarlet fever causes "scarlatina"—a fine, red, sandpaper-like rash with desquamation of the skin, commonly occurring during healing. "Strawberry tongue" commonly presents in the acute phase.

Streptococcal toxic shock syndrome (TSS) has gained attention lately. It causes symptoms similar to staphylococcal TSS (described below). Treatment is with IV penicillin (PCN), clindamycin +/- IVIG.

PCN is far and away the best treatment for a known group A strep throat infection. Give oral PCN (x 10 days) or IM benzathine PCN. Erythromycin for PCN-allergic. Clindamycin is often added to PCN when there is serious infection, such as necrotizing fasciitis or toxic shock.

Staphylococcus aureus

Impetigo. *S. aureus* is by far the most common cause of impetigo, which starts as an erythematous, vesicular lesion that quickly becomes pustular and crusty ("honey-colored crust"). Methicillin-resistant *Staphylococcus aureus* (MRSA) is the cause of many community outbreaks of impetigo. Treatment is covered in the Infectious Disease section.

Bullous impetigo usually occurs in young children < 2 years old and presents with the acute onset of large, loose bullae (Image 12-20).

Staphylococcal scalded skin syndrome (SSSS). Patients with SSSS present with tender, red, peeling skin—due to circulating toxins from localized staph infection or colonization, usually occurring at a non-skin site (sinuses; umbilicus in infants). Skin changes are similar to those seen in toxic epidermal necrolysis (noninfectious; rather, a side effect of drugs), so consider it during the workup. The skin in SSSS separates much more superficially than in toxic epidermal necrolysis (below)—through only the granular layer of the epidermis; therefore, SSSS is a much less serious disorder. (This separation is called a positive Nikolsky sign. Nikolsky sign is also seen in toxic epidermal necrolysis and pemphigus.)

Toxic shock syndrome (TSS). *S. aureus* and *S. pyogenes* are the causes of TSS. TSS presents with abrupt development of hypotension and multiorgan system failure. Patients have a diffuse scarlatiniform rash followed by desquamation of the palms and soles.

Staphylococcal scarlet fever can mimic streptococcal scarlet fever.

Furuncles and **folliculitis** are usually caused by *S. aureus*. Be aware that folliculitis associated with hot tub use is often caused by *Pseudomonas*, not staph.

Toxic epidermal necrolysis (TEN) is not a result of infection but is similar to SSSS (hence its mention here). It is considered a variant of Stevens-Johnson syndrome and is usually caused by a hypersensitivity reaction to a drug. Like SSSS, it results in a peeling or exfoliation of large areas of skin, but it occurs at a deeper level than SSSS. Patients with toxic epidermal necrolysis do poorly (mortality ~ 40%).

Gonococcus

Disseminated gonococcal infection causes a few (usually < 12) papular petechial lesions, which become pustular, often around the joints. Culture of disseminated exudate is usually negative. Culture is more sensitive when taken from the site of infection (cervix or urethra).

Meningococcemic skin signs start as macular or petechial lesions and evolve to large purpura.

Pseudomonas

Pseudomonas causes a variety of skin infections. It is the cause of "hot tub folliculitis." Normal chlorine levels may prevent the possibility or growth of infection with this organism. The pustules from hot tub folliculitis resolve without treatment in 1 week. Pseudomonal septicemia causes small, dark-centered (necrotic) papules. In a very

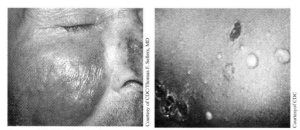

Image 12-19: Erysipelas   *Image 12-20: Bullous impetigo*

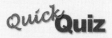

Quick Quiz

- What 2 organisms can cause impetigo?
- How does SSSS differ from toxic epidermal necrolysis?
- What do the lesions of disseminated gonococcal infection look like?
- Be able to recognize ecthyma gangrenosum and know what organism is responsible. Usually will see it in a febrile neutropenic patient!
- What agent is used to treat a cat bite?
- Molluscum contagiosum, if seen in an adult, should raise your suspicion for what immunodeficiency?

ill, neutropenic patient, this papule can evolve to ecthyma gangrenosum— a necrotic ulcer with an erythematous rim (Image 12-21).

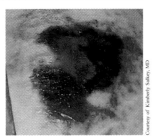

Image 12-21: Ecthyma gangrenosum

Animal Bites

S. aureus, *Eikenella*, and *Pasteurella multocida* often cause infection from dog and cat bites. Human bite infections are caused by multiple bacteria and can cause severe infection. Treatment: Clean and lavage well and give AM/CL (amoxicillin-clavulanate) as prophylaxis and treatment.

RICKETTSIAL SKIN INFECTIONS

Rocky Mountain spotted fever is usually heralded by several days of fever. Then the patient gets small lesions, which progress in distribution from peripheral to central and in type from macular to petechial to purpuric. As you can see from Image 12-22, the skin findings can be deceivingly nondescript.

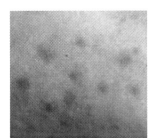

Image 12-22: Rocky Mountain spotted fever (medial foot)

SPIROCHETAL SKIN INFECTIONS

Lyme disease is often associated with erythema migrans (Image 12-23). This typically is a slowly (over about one week) enlarging annular erythematous rash with a clear center. Occasionally, the center will not be clear.

Syphilis. A chancre indicates primary syphilis. Diffuse scaling papules on the palms and soles, trunk, penis, and mucosal surfaces suggest secondary syphilis. Gummas occur in tertiary syphilis.

VIRAL SKIN INFECTIONS

Warts (verrucae) are caused by any one of more than 60 types of human papillomaviruses (HPV).

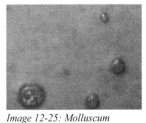

Image 12-23: Erythema migrans

- Verruca vulgaris is the common wart; you can treat it with liquid nitrogen, topical acids, CO_2 laser, etc.
- Verruca plana is the flat wart.
- Verruca plantaris is the plantar wart (Image 12-24). It is usually caused by HPV 1, 2, or 5. Initial treatment may consist of a strong acid (trichloroacetic acid), concentrated (40%) salicylic acid plaster, liquid nitrogen, or laser.
- Condyloma acuminata are anogenital warts. They are often caused by HPV 6 and 11. They are sometimes caused by HPV 16, 18, and 31—the HPVs associated with cancer of the cervix. You may treat them with podophyllin 25% in a tincture of benzoin, trichloroacetic acid, liquid nitrogen, or CO_2 laser. Podophyllin is teratogenic, so do not give it to pregnant patients. A newer treatment for condyloma acuminatum is topical imiquimod (Aldara®). HPV vaccine is recommended for all persons 9 to 26 years of age.

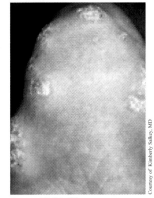

Image 12-24: Plantar wart

Molluscum contagiosum (Know) is caused by a Pox virus. It consists of smooth, umbilicated, pearly papules (Image 12-25). It usually occurs in children, but you may also see it in the pelvic area of sexually active young adults, and it is common in AIDS patients. It can be sexually transmitted in adults.

Image 12-25: Molluscum contagiosum

Measles (rubeola) has several stages. The prodromal stage lasts 3–4 days with fever, malaise, sinus discharge, and a hacking cough. Koplik spots often appear on the palate 1–2 days before the onset of rash. The red maculopapular rash starts on the forehead and quickly spreads

DERMATOLOGY

downward with the densest concentration of lesions from the forehead to the shoulders.

Rubella (German measles, 3-day measles) is benign except when it occurs in pregnant women. Congenital rubella results in a variety of serious birth defects: heart malformations, ocular defects, microcephaly, mental retardation, deafness, TTP, and bone problems.

Varicella-zoster virus (VZV) causes two diseases: chicken pox and herpes zoster (shingles). Herpes zoster is reactivation of VZV in a person who has had chickenpox.

Chicken pox: Only a minority of persons > age 15 are susceptible to infection. Rash is initially maculopapular and rapidly progresses to vesicles and then to scabbed lesions. These tend to come in "crops" over 2–4 days.

The herpes zoster skin manifestation is grouped vesicles along a dermatome. Topical acyclovir is not effective, although oral/IV acyclovir does help. Oral famciclovir and valacyclovir are also effective.

In the immunocompromised, you should treat both chicken pox and herpes zoster with intravenous acyclovir at higher doses than what is used to treat herpes simplex infections.

FUNGAL INFECTIONS

Tinea capitis (scalp ringworm), **tinea corporis** (common ringworm, Image 12-26), **tinea cruris** (jock itch—differential diagnosis includes moniliasis, which has satellite lesions), **tinea unguium** or **onychomycosis** (nails, Image 12-27), and **tinea pedis** (athlete's foot, Image 12-28).

Candidiasis of the mouth (thrush) causes white semi-adherent plaques on the tongue and mucosa. Vaginal candidiasis has similar plaques with cheesy discharge.

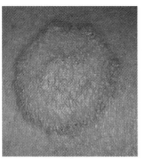

Image 12-26: Tinea corporis

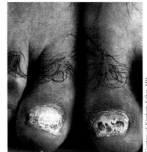

Image 12-27: Tinea unguium or onychomycosis

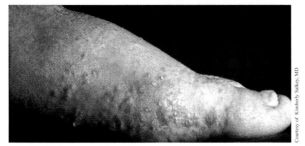

Image 12-28: Tinea pedis (athlete's foot)

Most fungal skin infections are controlled by topical antifungal creams. Miconazole, clotrimazole, and topical terbinafine (Lamisil®) are usually used. Tinea capitis requires oral therapy with griseofulvin, terbinafine, or itraconazole. Treat tinea unguium (onychomycosis) with systemic terbinafine, itraconazole, or fluconazole.

Tinea versicolor (Pityriasis versicolor) is caused by *Pityrosporum orbiculare* (also termed *Malassezia furfur*) (Image 12-29). Skin infection results in hypopigmented or hyperpigmented (depending on the patient's skin tone/color) spreading macules, usually on the upper torso and upper arms. Lesions do not fluoresce red with Wood's lamp as erythrasma does (page 12-7), although they may have yellowish fluorescence. KOH skin scraping: spaghetti and meatballs.

Treatment: imidazole creams, selenium sulfide or ketoconazole shampoo, and/or oral itraconazole.

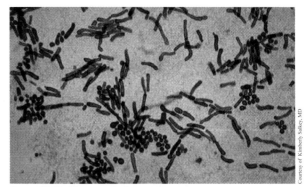

Image 12-29: Tinea versicolor

PARASITIC SKIN INFECTIONS

Lice (Pediculus humanus capitis/corporis): head or body louse. Phthirus pubis is the pubic louse ("crabs"). Outbreaks usually occur in schools, nursing home communities, and camps.

Head lice: The best pesticide-based topical treatment is over-the-counter permethrin cream 1% (Nix® cream rinse) because it kills both lice and eggs. It is approved for head lice only. The even more toxic topical medications, 1% lindane shampoo and pyrethrin + piperonyl butoxide (RID®, etc.), do not kill the eggs and require another treatment a week later. In the U.S., resistance is growing against all common pesticide-based preparations.

A newer treatment that is as effective as RID but contains no neurotoxic pesticides is benzyl alcohol lotion 5% (Ulesfia®). It kills by suffocating the lice. It is safe in children older than 6 months.

Malathion (topical) is the best prescription topical agent. Ivermectin (yes, the drug that kills heartworms in dogs; Stromectol®) is the strongest drug; it is given orally as 2 pills, 1 week apart. It is considered a 2nd line alternative to malathion.

Quick Quiz

- What are the treatments for head lice? What topical treatment is not pesticide-based?
- What is the metastatic potential for basal cell carcinoma?
- Squamous cell carcinoma has a high risk of metastatic transformation on which body parts?

Body lice (Image 12-30) live in clothes and are on the body only when feeding. Treatment is bathing and careful laundering of clothes and bed linens. 1% lindane lotion or pyrethrin + piperonyl butoxide are used if ova and/or parasites are found on the seams of clothing.

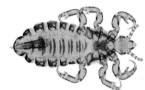

Pubic lice: The crab louse is sexually transmitted and can also infect the eyelashes. Crab lice are rarely

Image 12-30: Body louse

transmitted by fomites. Itching is the most common manifestation of infection. Exam may reveal bluish macules in the groin area. Treat with topical permethrin or pyrethrin + piperonyl butoxide. Wash bedding and clothing in hot water and use a hot dryer.

Scabies: is caused by a mite (*Sarcoptes scabiei*) that tunnels into the skin to lay eggs (Image 12-31). It is spread by skin-to-skin contact (will not live > 48 hours without a host!).

Treat with 5% permethrin applied to all areas of the body from the head down and washed off after 8 to 14 hours, or oral ivermectin with a repeat dose in 2 weeks. Lindane has CNS toxicity, so do not use it in infants and young children.

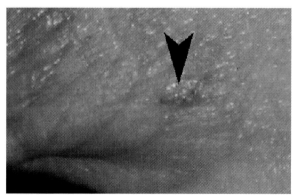

Image 12-31: Scabies tunnel

SKIN CANCER AND SKIN FINDINGS

Basal cell carcinoma (BCC): Arises from epidermal basal cells and is the most common form of skin cancer, especially in Caucasians (Image 12-32). The usual type of BCC is characterized by translucent pearly papules, often with telangiectatic vessels. It spreads by local extension and, when large enough, gets a "rodent-eaten" appearance.

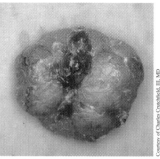

Image 12-32: Basal cell carcinoma

BCC is caused by ultraviolet (UV) radiation—from sun exposure. It is typically found on sun-exposed areas such as the head and neck, but it may appear elsewhere. UVA (320–400 nm) is the weakest type of UV light and is the type used in suntanning parlors, but it still can cause cancer. UVB (290–320 nm) is the cause of sunburn and is 1,000x more erythemogenic than UVA.

Know that the metastatic potential of BCC is < 0.1%.

Squamous cell carcinoma (SCC): From keratinizing epidermal cells, SCC occurs especially in fair-skinned persons and on exposed areas, like the dorsum of hands, forearms, ears, and lower lip (Image 12-33). It has several associated precancerous lesions, especially actinic keratosis. In contrast to the low metastatic potential of BCC, SCC has a 0.3–3.7% metastatic potential—and even higher when it appears on the ear (11%) and lower lip (13%)! Metastatic rate of recurring tumors is 30%.

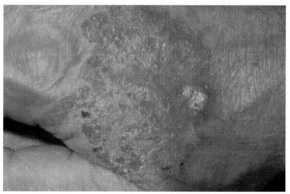

Image 12-33: Squamous cell carcinoma of the hand

Melanoma: Also tends to occur more commonly in fair-skinned people, especially those who had severe sunburn in childhood (Image 12-34). There has been a 300% increase in the past 40 years. Other risk factors are dysplastic nevus (described below), family history of melanoma, a high number of ordinary melanotic nevi, a congenital melanotic nevus, and immunosuppression. It is almost always completely curable if caught early enough.

DERMATOLOGY

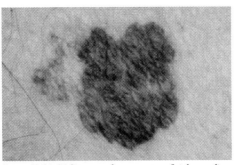

Image 12-34: Malignant melanoma—superficial spreading

Think "ABCDE" when assessing a lesion that might be malignant melanoma:

A: asymmetry; B: borders are irregular; C: colors are variable; D: diameter > 5 mm is suspicious; and E: elevated or evolving lesions are more suspicious.

Age of the patient, location of the lesion, and (most important) depth of the lesion are prognostic factors.

Age < 50 and location on the trunk are better prognostic factors.

Lesions < 0.76 mm in depth have a 99% five-year survival; those > 3.6 mm have a < 50% five-year survival. If the lesion is < 0.76 mm, you may safely excise the melanoma with a 1 cm tumor-free margin (previously a 5 cm margin was recommended).

Dysplastic nevi are "odd-looking" moles and may even look like melanomas (Image 12-35). They are markers for propensity to develop malignant melanoma. Most melanomas arise de novo. Removing all the moles does not prevent melanoma development. Standard of care is close follow-up and monitoring, utilizing photographic documentation. If a patient with a dysplastic nevus has two relatives with malignant melanoma, the patient has a 300x chance of getting malignant melanoma!

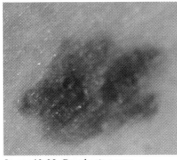

Image 12-35: Dysplastic nevus

Sézary syndrome and **mycosis fungoides** are the main forms of cutaneous T-cell lymphoma. Sézary syndrome has peripheral blood involvement and poorer prognosis.

Paget disease of the breast is something you should consider anytime there is a persistent (despite treatment), unilateral, oozing, eczematous plaque in the area of the areola. It is virtually always due to underlying breast cancer. By far, the most common cause of an acute eczema-type rash on an areola is just a contact dermatitis or skin irritation. Consider Paget disease only if there is no response to treatment.

Peutz-Jeghers syndrome consists of multiple hamartomatous polyps + melanotic pigmentation (lentigines) on the lips + buccal mucosa. Even though these polyps are hamartomas, there is still some risk of cancer because an occasional adenoma will occur. Note that healthy, darkly pigmented people and those with Addison disease may have similar intraoral dark spots.

Sweet syndrome is also called acute febrile neutrophilic dermatosis. Patients have high fever and painful red plaques, ~ 1 inch in diameter. A skin biopsy shows a dense neutrophilic infiltrate. 10% or less are associated with leukemia (AML and myelomonocytic leukemia are the most common). Corticosteroids are usually quickly effective.

Glucagonomas (secreting pancreatic alpha cell tumors) can cause a beefy red tongue (think GLucagonoma = GLossitis), angular cheilitis, and a necrolytic migratory erythematous rash. Patients with glucagonomas typically develop the "four Ds": diabetes, DVT, depression, and dermatitis.

The 4 cancers that most commonly have cutaneous metastases are lung cancer, GI cancer, melanoma, and breast cancer in women.

Macroglossia associated with pinch purpura, which develops from pinching or stroking the skin, strongly suggests multiple myeloma and/or cutaneous amyloidosis.

BLISTERING LESIONS

Porphyria cutanea tarda (PCT) (Image 12-36, Image 12-37) is the most common type of porphyria. PCT causes hyperpigmentation and tense blisters in sun-exposed areas, milia, skin fragility, and increased facial hair. Porphyria is caused by a congenital or acquired decreased activity of uroporphyrinogen decarboxylase, which allows a buildup of phototoxic porphyrins in the skin. Symptoms can be induced by ingestion of estrogen or alcohol! Many patients have associated hepatitis C. Lab

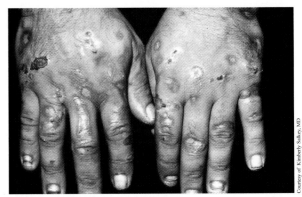

Image 12-36: Porphyria cutanea tarda (PCT)

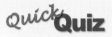
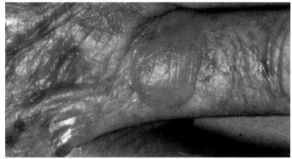

Image 12-37: Porphyria cutanea tarda (PCT) with blisters

results usually show an increased serum Fe, HCT, ALT, and AST. To screen, check for increased urinary copro-porphyrins and uroporphyrins. Patients may have dark or pink urine. Treatment is the same as for hemochromatosis: regular phlebotomies. Antimalarials may also help. PCT due to HCV resolves with treatment of hepatitis.

Porphyria variegata (variegate porphyria) is also known as South African porphyria. Patients may get blisters on sun-exposed areas and have mechanical fragility of the skin. These patients may also have abdominal pain, poly-neuropathies, and mental disturbances. Treatment of acute attacks is the same as for acute intermittent porphyria (AIP): glucose and hematin. Differential diagnosis: Note that AIP presents similarly to variegate porphyria, except without the skin changes. PCT (above) presents with the skin changes and without the neuro/mental changes!

Epidermolysis bullosa: Patients have blistering after minor skin trauma, caused by congenital structural defects of the skin. There are many different classifications. It is genetically transmitted.

Epidermolysis bullosa acquisita, like bullous pemphigoid (next), is also caused by antibodies directed against the basement membrane. The target antigen is type VII collagen.

Bullous pemphigoid causes recurrent crops of tense blisters (Image 12-38). It has an autoimmune etiology.

There are anti-basement membrane antibodies, although it is unclear what the specific target antigen is. Treatment is primarily topical steroids.

Pemphigus vulgaris (Image 12-39) probably has a multifactorial etiology with a common autoimmune result—an antibody against the desmosomal proteins. This causes acantholysis (the separation of epidermal cells from each other

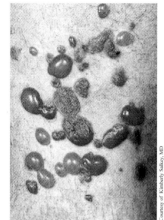

Image 12-38: Bullous pemphigoid

due to decreased cohesion), which results in the formation of large, loose bullae that peel off and leave denuded skin. Oral mucosal involvement is common, and any cutaneous area can be affected.

Treat pemphigus vulgaris with high-dose corticosteroids +/– cyclosporine/azathioprine/cyclophosphamide and IVIG.

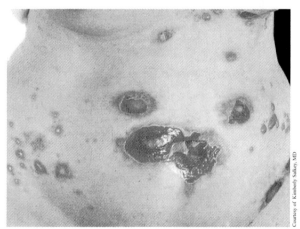

Image 12-39: Pemphigus vulgaris

Nikolsky sign is epidermal sliding with digital pressure on the skin and indicates the acantholysis that causes the symptoms. (Nikolsky sign is also seen in toxic epidermal necrolysis and staphylococcal scalded skin syndrome [SSSS]).

Erythema multiforme consists of well-defined lesions varying from annular to target shape (Image 12-40). Palms and soles are frequently involved, and mucous membranes may be affected. The target- or iris-shaped lesions are pathognomonic for erythema multiforme. The lesions may also be edematous or bullous. It is caused by drugs and many infectious and noninfectious diseases.

Herpes simplex is a common predisposing condition for erythema multiforme, and treatment for herpes simplex can sometimes cure recurrent erythema

DERMATOLOGY

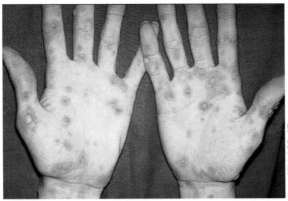

Image 12-40: Erythema multiforme

multiforme. *Mycoplasma* infection is a common bacterial precondition.

Erythema multiforme can be confused with photosensitive side effects of medications. Rule these out first. Commonly implicated drugs are thiazides, tetracycline, phenothiazine, sulfonamides, quinolones, and piroxicam (Feldene®).

Stevens-Johnson syndrome is a severe form of erythema multiforme, and some authors consider it part of the spectrum of toxic epidermal necrolysis (TEN). Corticosteroids are controversial and should be used for only a very short time, if at all.

Dermatitis herpetiformis is a skin disease where very pruritic vesicular lesions appear, usually on the extensor surfaces and mid- to lower back, caused by IgA deposition (Image 12-41). It is associated with celiac disease (gluten-sensitive enteropathy).

ROUND LESIONS

Granuloma annulare is an annular, ringworm-like lesion without scaling, which usually appears on the distal portion of the extremities (Image 12-42). It often occurs in children and young women. It usually is self-limited, disappearing in months to a few years.

Nummular eczema consists of small, circular (nummular = coin-shaped) lesions that are more common on the lower legs and are often associated with dry skin

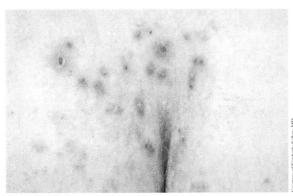

Image 12-41: Dermatitis herpetiformis

and atopy. They are very common in the elderly and have no pathologic significance. Rule out fungal infection.

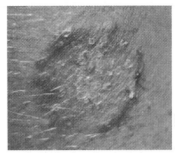

Image 12-42: Granuloma annulare

Pityriasis rosea is a rash you see especially in children and young adults. It probably has a viral etiology (possibly human herpesvirus 6 or 7). The disease is self-limited, usually lasting 4–8 weeks.

A herald patch precedes subsequent lesions by 1–2 weeks (Image 12-43). This patch is sometimes confused with tinea corporus (Image 12-26 on page 12-10). It develops into small, pruritic papulosquamous oval lesions with the long axis parallel to skin folds and rib lines in a "Christmas tree" pattern (Image 12-44). Treatment is symptomatic. Note that tinea versicolor (= pityriasis versicolor) has no relationship with pityriasis rosea.

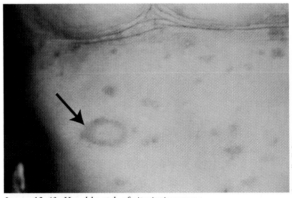

Image 12-43: Herald patch of pityriasis rosea

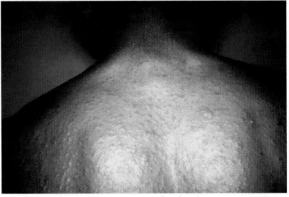

Image 12-44: Pityriasis rosea; generalized rash

PIGMENT CHANGES

Vitiligo is an autoimmune, spreading, macular depigmentation (Image 12-45). It usually occurs in healthy persons, but, rarely, it may also be part of the autosomal recessive polyglandular deficiency. With this, there may be any

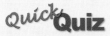

Quick Quiz

- Which virus is often responsible for erythema multiforme?
- What GI disorder is dermatitis herpetiformis associated with?
- What is characterized by a "Christmas tree" pattern and a herald patch?
- What skin finding might you see in an autosomal recessive polyglandular deficiency?
- Hyperpigmented areas of the axilla are usually due to what?
- What virus causes oral hairy leukoplakia in AIDS patients?

of the following: DM, Graves disease, Addison disease/ adrenal insufficiency, hyper- or hypothyroidism, hypoparathyroidism, and pernicious anemia. Anytime you see a patient with vitiligo, think of these possibilities!

Tuberous sclerosis is uncommon and autosomal dominant. It is associated with seizures, mental retardation, periungual fibromas, and hypopigmented (ash-leaf) macules. You will see these macules best with a Wood's lamp. Adenoma sebaceum manifests in these patients as numerous mid-facial papules, which are actually angiofibromas.

Café-au-lait spots are brown macules that occur in association with neurofibromatosis (von Recklinghausen disease) and Albright disease but also, to a lesser degree, in people with no disease (1–2 spots are normal and common). In neurofibromatosis, 78% of patients have > 6 spots—and 95% have at least one spot > 1.5 cm. In Albright disease, the spots have a more irregular outline.

Acanthosis nigricans is hyperpigmented skin with a thickened, velvety appearance, most noticed in the skin folds (Image 12-46). Involvement of the axilla is usually shown as an example. It rarely is familial.

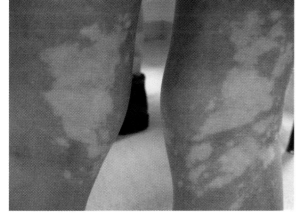

Image 12-45: Vitiligo

Although you will usually see this in obese patients, it is also associated with GI cancer, many endocrinopathies, and several autoimmune problems. The malignant acanthosis nigricans is severe and progressive and is usually associated with gastric adenocarcinoma. Associated endocrinopathies include Cushing disease, hyper/ hypothyroidism, acromegaly, and diabetes mellitus. Overuse of niacin may also cause acanthosis nigricans!

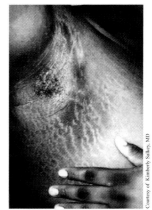

Image 12-46: Acanthosis nigricans

Diffuse hyperpigmentation may occur in biliary sclerosis, scleroderma, Addison disease, hemochromatosis (a grayish/bronze coloration), and with the use of the cancer drug busulfan. Other causes include primary biliary cirrhosis, porphyria cutanea tarda, malabsorption and/or Whipple syndrome, pellagra (niacin deficiency), B_{12} deficiency, and folate deficiency. Check for metastatic melanoma in "slate-blue" patients!

Hyperpigmentation in sun-exposed areas: amiodarone, porphyria cutanea tarda, phenothiazines. Hyperpigmentation is diffuse but darker in sun-exposed areas in pellagra, biliary sclerosis, and scleroderma. Methotrexate can cause a reactivation of sunburn.

Black lesions. Consider the following when you see black lesions:

- Rhinocerebral mucormycosis
- Anthrax
- Ecthyma gangrenosum
- Emboli into distal extremities
- Melanoma/lentigo
- Warfarin skin necrosis
- Glucagonomas causing necrolytic dermatitis

PRURITUS

The most common cause of itching in elderly patients is dry skin. Other causes seen across the age spectrum include:

- Hyper- or hypothyroidism
- Malignancy: think lymphoma—especially Hodgkin's, but also breast cancer
- Fe deficiency (even if patient is not anemic)
- Chronic (but not acute) renal failure, commonly treated with ultraviolet B phototherapy or activated charcoal
- Cholestatic liver disease

AIDS-RELATED SKIN LESIONS

AIDS-related lesions include the following: xerosis (dry skin), seborrheic dermatitis (in virtually all patients!), telangiectasias, herpes simplex, herpes zoster, folliculitis, Kaposi sarcoma (KS), and oral candidiasis. Patients with HIV/AIDS can also get condyloma acuminatum, molluscum contagiosum, and bacillary angiomatosis. Bacillary angiomatosis resembles KS but is caused by a gram-negative bacillus similar to the one that causes cat scratch fever.

Treat the seborrheic dermatitis with topical low-potency steroids +/– an antifungal shampoo.

The folliculitis is usually due to uncontrolled HIV infection, but it can also be due to a yeast, *Pityrosporum orbiculare,* or *Staphylococcus aureus*. Usually antiretroviral treatment improves these rashes.

Oral "hairy" leukoplakia (Image 12-9 on page 12-3) is a corrugated tongue with white lesions along the side. You see it virtually only in patients with HIV infection. Epstein-Barr virus is the cause. It resolves with treatment of HIV.

Kaposi sarcoma is usually seen as < 0.5 cm purple/red/violet macular/papular lesions. They are usually oval with a long axis along skin folds (like pityriasis rosea) and occur anywhere on the body.

Herpes zoster is often refractory to treatment in these patients. Treat with acyclovir or famciclovir. Valacyclovir has been associated with thrombotic thrombocytopenic purpura in the immunocompromised, so isn't recommended.

Disseminated *Cryptococcus* infection may imitate molluscum contagiosum.

DIABETIC SKIN LESIONS

Diabetes-associated skin lesions include eruptive xanthomas due to hypertriglyceridemia. Eruptive xanthomas are usually an indication that the diabetes is out of control. These lesions will resolve when the hyperglycemia is controlled (Image 12-47).

Necrobiosis lipoidica diabeticorum, as the name suggests, is associated with diabetes in 75% of cases (Image 12-48). It is a thin, atrophic, vascular plaque that appears on the shins. It is subject to trauma and ulceration and is thought to be due to microangiopathy.

Diabetic skin spots (diabetic dermopathy) are dark atrophic macules; they are common and often appear on the shins. They have no clinical significance.

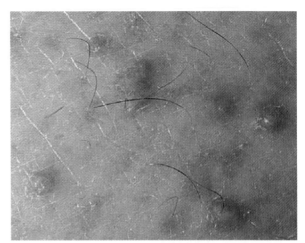
Image 12-47: Eruptive xanthomas in a diabetic

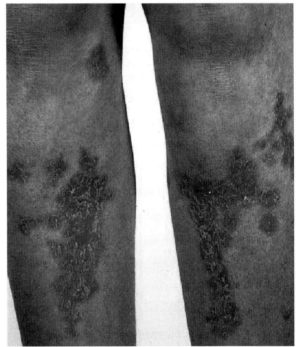
Image 12-48: Necrobiosis lipoidica diabeticorum

Courtesy of Kimberly Salkey, MD

NOTES